THE
SELF-HEALING
PERSONALITY

Why Some People Achieve Health
and Others Succumb to Illness

Dr. Howard S. Friedman

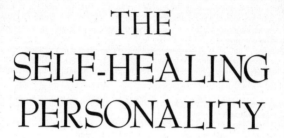

A PLUME BOOK

Note

An important note to our readers. This book was written to educate and inform, and to enable you to understand the nature of health and health care. The book is not designed to advise or instruct you as to specifically what must be done in a particular case. It is wise to consult with a doctor before undertaking an exercise program, changing your diet, or taking any medication.

For case histories of self-healing and disease-prone personalities reported in this book, names and identifying details have been altered to protect the individuals' identities.

PLUME
Published by the Penguin Group
Penguin Books USA Inc., 375 Hudson Street, New York, New York 10014, U.S.A.
Penguin Books Ltd, 27 Wrights Lane, London W8 5TZ, England
Penguin Books Australia Ltd, Ringwood, Victoria, Australia
Penguin Books Canada Ltd, 10 Alcorn Avenue, Toronto, Ontario, Canada M4V 3B2
Penguin Books (N.Z.) Ltd, 182-190 Wairau Road, Auckland 10, New Zealand

Penguin Books Ltd, Registered Offices: Harmondsworth, Middlesex, England

Published by Plume, an imprint of New American Library, a division of Penguin Books USA Inc. This is an authorized reprint of a hardcover edition published by Henry Holt and Company, Inc.

First Plume Printing, February, 1992
10 9 8 7 6 5 4 3 2 1

 REGISTERED TRADEMARK—MARCA REGISTRADA

LIBRARY OF CONGRESS CATALOGING-IN-PUBLICATION DATA
Friedman, Howard S.
   The self-healing personality : why some people achieve health and
others succumb to illness / Howard S. Friedman.
      p.   cm.
   Originally published: New York : H. Holt, 1991.
   Includes bibliographical references and index.
   ISBN 0-452-26757-9
   1. Clinical health psychology. 2. Medicine, Psychosomatic.
I. Title.
[R726.7.F754   1992]
616'.001'9—dc20   91-36560
                                                              CIP

Printed in the United States of America
Original hardcover design by Katy Riegel

To my wife, Miriam Schustack,
whose love promotes my health

Contents

Preface   ix

Acknowledgments   xi

1. The Challenge of Healing   1

2. How Can Personality Be Related to Health?   13

3. Stress: Our Current Understanding   30

4. Negative Emotions and Health   45

5. Disease-prone Personalities   57

6. Personalities That Resist Disease:
    The Self-healing Personality   98

7. Inner Healing Through Nerves and Hormones   129

8. Achieving Homeostasis: Developing a
    Self-healing Personality   154

9. Is There a Health Conspiracy? What Can Society Do?
    What Will Future Research Bring?   202

    Notes   221

    Index   233

Preface

The decade of the 1990s will see dramatic changes in our understanding of physical health and healing. Major scientific breakthroughs are showing current medical perspectives to be sadly inadequate. Attention is turning to the unique reaction patterns of the *individual*.

Many pieces of the puzzle of a new view of health have now been uncovered. The overall picture is waiting to be discerned. In this book, I have endeavored to place the fragments into a recognizable pattern that reveals why some people achieve health while others succumb to illness.

I would like to note the special contributions of my editor, the late Donald Hutter, for having had faith that this book could maintain high scientific standards while reaching a wide audience.

—Howard S. Friedman
San Diego, California

Acknowledgments

My seven-year-long study of personality, emotions, and health has taken me in many directions and depended on the insights of many people. I have a chance here to acknowledge only a few:

My staff, students, and colleagues at the University of California campuses have always supported my striking out in new directions. A number of my students have provided helpful suggestions or insights, especially Merril Bedrin, Patty Hawley, Bo Josephson, Dr. Barbara Keesling, Dr. Stephanie Kewley, Joan Tucker, and Mamie Wong. Professor Robert Rosenthal of Harvard University has supported my scientific career in innumerable ways. Friends and family who shared their reactions to my early drafts include Ellen Finan, Norma and Norman Goldberg, Matt Greenberg, Dan Schustack, Dr. Miriam Schustack, and Madeline Taylor. My literary agent, Barbara Lowenstein, got me going, full steam ahead. Finally, the people at Henry Holt and Company were always helpful, professional, and supportive.

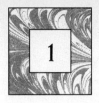

The Challenge of Healing

Modern health care has not kept up with the reality of present-day threats to health. Most illnesses of our times—heart disease, stroke, cancer, diabetes, asthma, ulcers, arthritis—are not primarily communicable afflictions brought on by sudden infection. Rather, they are slowly developing chronic conditions that many men and women can prevent or conquer. However, the individual must take an active role to maintain health and to recover from illness.

I have never seen a death certificate marked "Death due to unhealthy personality." But maybe pathologists and coroners should be instructed to take into account the latest scientific findings on the role of personality in health. Personality affects our susceptibility to disease, and there are ways we can improve our odds for good health.

I have never heard someone being told, "You are too mellow and relaxed; to remain healthy, you really should develop some stresses and neuroses." No one contends that happy people are at higher risk for developing a crippling or fatal disease. Instead we hear that chronic worriers tend to get ulcers and that headaches may be the result of a hostile character. People with cancer may be accused of having a repressed personality and of thereby damaging their own health. Heart attacks? Almost everyone seems to believe that they are at least partly due to having a workaholic-type personality.

Is an emotionally troubled person really at higher risk for developing a crippling or fatal condition? What does the scientific evidence say, and what can we do about it? I first asked myself these questions about a decade ago, while at work in my laboratory at the University of California conducting videotape studies of how people express emotions. I found that not everyone would or could express emotions freely and truly. For example, one young woman I studied appeared disgusted while she *claimed* to be feeling happy and seductive. (Needless to say, she was not very successful with members of the opposite sex.) Anxious and pessimistic, she frequently suffered from allergies, migraines, and dizziness.

Other people I studied appeared generally hostile, others were sad, and still others showed no emotion whatsoever. These individual differences in emotional expressions seemed closely related to personality. People had characteristic modes of expression.

At about the same time, I was writing a book about the fast-developing field called health psychology. I kept running across scientific references to people whose hurried and active emotional style seemed to predispose them to heart disease. Many of these hurried people sounded exactly like certain people I had been studying—individuals who were fast-moving, dominant, and hyper-alert, but not at all unhealthy! On the contrary, they were exceptionally healthy, both physically and mentally. As I became more and more puzzled, I began to examine the matter in greater and greater detail.

My search led me back in time to read and reanalyze older, forgotten studies of personality, emotions, and health, and it led me to evaluate current research and to design new studies of my own. I was amazed at what I found. Most researchers had little knowledge of what other researchers were doing, and it seemed as if many of them were missing the forest for the trees. I decided to tackle the task of pulling it all together.

I began with a list of diseases that are commonly believed to be related to psychological state—asthma, arthritis, ulcers, headaches, and heart disease. As my work developed, I added cancer and other disorders to the list. I first asked two simple questions: Are these diseases reliably found to be associated with emotional states, such as anxiety, hostility, or depression? If so, are the same emotions relevant to the different diseases?

Inexplicably, these issues had not been systematically addressed in more than a generation. The field called *psychosomatic medicine* had nearly collapsed in the 1950s, almost disgraced by exaggerated claims. My questions rapidly became more and more sophisticated as I was forced to define emotional disturbance, trace physiological links, and quantify the nature of the associations to illness. I began using newly refined statistical techniques called *meta-analyses*, which allow the statistical combination of the results of hundreds of studies. I was surprised and pleased with what I found. Piecing together research results from many different domains, I uncovered fascinating indications of who would resist disease and who would likely succumb. This book reports the results of my scientific expedition.

So again, is an emotionally troubled person really at higher risk for developing a crippling or fatal condition? The new analyses of old studies coupled with new research breakthroughs strongly suggest that yes, there is indeed a healing personality and a corresponding disease-prone personality, *but many commonly held conceptions are in error*.

While some have claimed that we can use our minds to build up our immunities and "will" our way to health, there is good reason to doubt whether such a process is generally effective. Although there is some truth to such claims, they are only part of the story. Many people try to "think positive" but still find themselves in poor health, and many other people are simply unable to maintain a smiling face and cheery disposition—they get anxious, angry, depressed, or tense. Still others, however, do manage to play a positive role in their own well-being. In other words, there are tremendous differences among individuals.

INDIVIDUAL DIFFERENCES

Doctors are continually amazed at how two people with similar medical conditions can respond so differently. After an operation for breast cancer, one woman feels fine and goes on to lead a healthy life, while a second woman with a similar tumor quickly succumbs to the cancer. Some people seem prone to all types of health problems, while others rarely get sick. These differences remain even after we take into account obvious differences among people, such as whether one is a chain-smoker. There is something about certain individuals that protects their health.

Hard work and constant business demands are stressful and unhealthy for some people. Yet other people stay healthy and even thrive in demanding situations. These differences are enhanced when there is an existing medical condition. For example, some diabetics show a dangerous increase in blood sugar when stressed, but other diabetics do not.

People have different temperaments, face different challenges, and employ different coping skills. Perhaps a Zen master can harmonize the body through deep meditation; not everyone can be a Zen master.

Ronald Reagan was a healthy, active president at age seventy-seven. He survived both a serious gunshot wound and colon cancer to continue working at one of the most demanding jobs in the world. He remained a popular and influential leader well into old age.

Many other people of prominence have led active and productive lives well beyond age seventy. Eleanor Roosevelt and Benjamin Franklin made major contributions to world affairs late in life. Was this commitment to a better world relevant to their health? Bob Hope, George Burns, and other comedians have entertained millions of people when in their eighties. In an interview, Hope claimed that telling jokes "helps your stomach, helps your everything." Does it? Can it work for everyone?

Vladimir Horowitz, Pablo Casals, and many other musicians and performers seemed to go on and on, well into old age. Not only could these performers continue working late in life, but they retained that magical spark and joie de vivre that audiences find so appealing. Jonas Salk, Benjamin Spock, Margaret Mead, and many other scientists have contributed important ideas at an old age. One's intellectual capacity does not necessarily decline.

Contrary to public opinion, it is not "natural" for most people to become decrepit by their sixties. For many people who die of heart disease in their fifties or cancer in their sixties, it is a distortion to list the death as due to "natural causes." Most could have lived a longer and healthier life. Those who live to a healthy old age differ in systematic ways from those who succumb.

The longevity of extraordinary people like Bob Hope and Benjamin Franklin is not in itself scientific proof of anything. However, the personalities of these people provide insights into and illustrations of the findings that have emerged from scientific research. The scientific evidence for the role of personality in maintaining health has appeared only in the last few years. But the basic idea dates back thousands of years.

MEDICINE AND THE INDIVIDUAL PERSONALITY

Hippocrates, the ancient Greek father of medicine, must have been an interesting character. Rebelling against the idea that health was a function of gods and demons, he began the scientific study of health, both physical and mental. Hippocrates described four basic bodily fluids, or "humors," as the basis of personality. These were extended by the physician Galen and others to apply directly to physical as well as mental health. Their scheme of humors and humoral disturbances dominated medicine for almost two thousand years.

Galen, a Greek who wrote in Roman times, was trained as a philosopher as well as a physician. Perhaps it was his philosophical training that led him to think especially deeply about the individual's position in the world. It is interesting to note that his name, Galenos, means calm, serene, or mild in Greek. As we shall see, both Galen's ancient medicine and the most modern understanding of the nature of health emphasize a type of serenity and the avoidance of extremes.

The four bodily humors were said to be blood, black bile (or melancholy), yellow bile (or choler), and phlegm. A dominance of blood led to a sanguine and ruddy person. Too much black bile meant proneness to depression and degenerative disease. The yellow bile supposedly caused the angry (choleric), bitter personality. Phlegm was the cold and moist humor, said to cause apathy.

Unfortunately, physicians and other healers tried to influence these humors directly to cure the sick. Efforts to restore humoral balance led to bleedings, purgings, and other bodily invasions, many of them fatal. Bloodletting was prescribed for everything from coughs to flatulence.

In 1799, George Washington was bled of several pints of blood and was given a drink to induce vomiting and diarrhea. He died soon thereafter.

Modern physiologists never would search the body for humors; they look for chemical transmitters in the brain and hormones in the blood. But even though the search for humoral balance has been thoroughly discredited, the four emotional aspects of personality that so influenced medical practice for two thousand years—cheerfulness, depression, hostility, and apathy—remain the key ones for understanding personality and health today. The ancient Greeks were on the right track.

Consider, for example, the case of a patient named Agnes, an unhappy and unattractive woman of fifty who had a serious heart condition that her doctors had labeled "cause unknown." Agnes had been in and out of hospitals, but no physician could help her. She finally died in the hospital on her birthday; she had always wanted to show her resentment at being born.

Agnes was not a patient of the 1990s but a patient of the 1930s. She was described by Dr. Flanders Dunbar in a classic book about psychosomatic medicine. Dunbar discovered that Agnes had grown up in a hateful environment, with her mother constantly reminding her that Agnes was a mistake—the mother had never wanted a child. Dr. Dunbar's point was that such stresses would inevitably end up "with the outraged emotional system taking its revenge upon the body in the form of a disease which physicians will be able to recognize but not cure."

Such cases are still common. Several years ago, I went to consult with one of the world's leading cardiologists. Top physicians from all over the world come to study in this cardiologist's lab and learn the latest and the best in cardiac care. This is also the kind of place that physicians themselves go when they think they have a serious heart problem. This cardiologist and professor, wiser than most, made sure to emphasize to his students the psychological influences on physical health.

During one seminar, he described the case of a woman who had been referred to him after other cardiologists could not diagnose her unusual heart abnormalities. The medical fellows in the seminar suggested all sorts of fancy tests and diagnoses, many of them quite insightful; but none correctly identified the woman's problem. It turned out that she was a religious woman with nine children and was looking for a doctor who would tell her that she needed to be sterilized. She was seeking the medical stamp of approval for a solution to her social and relational problems.

EXPECTATIONS AND HEALTH

Every few years, a controversial new miracle drug makes headlines as a supposed cure for a dreaded disease. The scientific community warns that the drug has not been proven effective in controlled clinical trials, while the drug's proponents argue that ill and dying victims of disease are being deprived of their sole hope for survival.

My favorite case involves the supposed anticancer drug named Krebiozen, popular in the 1950s. This case is particularly interesting because the appearance and use of Krebiozen was paralleled in almost exact form two decades later by the drug Laetrile. Krebiozen, a derivative of the blood serum of horses, created a panic in the early 1950s as word leaked out that it could cure cancer. Desperate patients tried any means to get the new treatment. Cancer patients given the drug felt better, had less pain, and often lived longer than expected. In some cases, tumors shrank dramatically. But no scientific study could ever show its effectiveness, and it was banned by the Food and Drug Administration, much to the chagrin of many patients.

Laetrile, extracted from apricot pits, had been kicking around the fringes of the medical community for many years. But in the 1970s it suddenly made a dramatic appearance, with emotional testimonials as to its curative powers. Cancer patients again flocked to secret clinics, this time for Laetrile. The actor Steve McQueen, dying of cancer, made much-publicized visits to Mexico for Laetrile treatment. This drug was never found to have any scientific effectiveness, but everyone knew the drug sometimes "worked." Again there were charges of a medical coverup, congressional hearings, and much public controversy.

How can the success of these substances be explained? The power of Krebiozen and Laetrile was a sort of faith healing. It was a faith healing that really worked . . . for some people.

In the general prologue to *The Canterbury Tales*, Chaucer tells us that with the arrival of spring, "then longen folk to go on pilgrimages . . . The holy blissful martyr for to seek, that them hath helped when that they were sick." The martyr was Archbishop Thomas à Becket, who had been murdered in Canterbury. The archbishop's blood, saved by his associates, was soon recognized for its tremendous healing powers.

In the twentieth century, European pilgrims are more likely to visit Lourdes, France. The visit is a very emotional one. Thousands of chronic invalids gather, and most feel better afterward even though they are not cured. However, over the years, many people have been cured, at least partly, at Lourdes, as a pile of discarded crutches attests. Interestingly, the cured patients report feeling a tremendous sense of serenity and goodwill. Unfortunately, such so-called placebo effects— the power of faith and belief—are often terribly misunderstood.

Thousands of such cases of miracle cures have been documented in the medical literature. There is no doubt that they exist, even though they often are ignored in routine health care. Psychological and emotional factors, often reportedly involving some kind of divine inspiration, affect our physical health. Anyone who has done any reading on the topic has heard this asserted again and again. We do not need more examples. Case studies of miraculous recoveries are not strong scientific evidence. What we do need is a comprehensive understanding of such phenomena that takes into account the latest scientific findings on personality and health.

Although not directly harmful, Krebiozen and Laetrile do indeed inflict harm. They lead cancer patients away from treatments that are valid and more effective and they waste a lot of money. Patients, dissatisfied with their doctors, may travel from clinic to clinic or even drop out of the health care system entirely, seeking quack cures. Thus, ironically, these worthless drugs really do have some worth: they remind us that psychosocial factors are a crucial aspect of health and that such factors, when ignored by our traditional health care system, lead us to incur large costs.

HEALING OUR HEALTH CARE SYSTEM

As any health economist, financial executive, or patient paying health insurance premiums well knows, health care costs are astronomical. It is not an exaggeration to say that the traditional fee-for-service health care system is going broke. In the United States, well over 10 percent of the gross national product is spent on health care, and costs grow every year. Everyone who examines these phenomenal costs knows that something has to give, something has to change. In many countries (including Canada and most of Europe), the change has been to government-controlled medical care.

Paradoxically, at the same time that more and more money is being spent, patients and health care personnel in the United States are less and less satisfied. Patients grumble about uncaring doctors, complain about limited access to health services, and sue for malpractice. Nurses have left their profession in droves. Physicians suffer with high malpractice insurance premiums, governmental and organizational intrusion into their practices, and unhappy patients. These problems are all symptoms that something has gone drastically wrong with our understanding of health and health care.

As health care costs continue to skyrocket during the next decade, a health revolution will begin to brew. Dramatic changes will occur. These changes have already hit indigent people. The poor have either very little health care or health care that is strictly regulated by the government. The government decides how much it will pay and what it will pay for; doctors and hospitals then apportion the limited resources accordingly. The American middle classes are about to get hit. Insurance premiums and deductibles will rise, while freedom of medical choice will decline. Sadly, the coming crunch could be, but probably will not be, headed off.

Why are we spending more money on health care and getting poor results? Although the details are complicated, the essence of the answer is simple: We are using an outdated model of health and illness that does not fit current realities.

THE TEN THOUSAND–MILE SERVICE
AND THE ANNUAL PHYSICAL

In modern Western societies, medical care systems are built around a traditional model of disease that resembles our view of automobile engines. Human bodies are seen as either "healthy" running machines or as breakdowns. When your body breaks down, you go to a doctor and have a part replaced, a valve repaired, or a general exam and tune-up. Although this approach sometimes leads to wonderful medical miracles, it ignores the realities of the basic threats to health in modern societies.

A heart transplant operation can cost $150,000 or more. This figure does not include the patient's lost wages, long-term rehabilitation costs, or many costs of the health care infrastructure. Despite the costs, such patients have a good chance of dying either during the operation or within a few years following the procedure. Is it worth it? If we are the patient or the spouse of the patient who is about to die without the transplant, we probably are inclined to think that the operation is worth it.

Consider now the case of coronary artery bypass operations, which threaten to become as common as engine overhauls in automobiles, even though they are very costly and fairly risky. Clogged arteries are a major health problem. As our population gets older, more and more people suffer from this condition. Also, the relevant medical technology continues to become more and more sophisticated. Not only can we transplant the engine, we can rewire it, clean it, and tune it, and we can replace the drive shaft, the windows, and the tires.

In my grade school of the 1950s, there was a full-time nurse, and the school district had a physician. All of my classmates were fully immunized against contagious diseases to the extent that vaccines were available. The social structure relevant to health was different, too. For example, grandparents lived near their grown children, and when the old folks became too frail, they often lived with their children. Heart transplants and coronary bypass operations were not available.

It would be easy to fill in many more details concerning the family doctor, the clean water, the neighborhood community, and so on. This is not to say that the 1950s were perfect or that there have not been tremendous medical breakthroughs during the past forty years. On the contrary: in the past, heart disease was usually fatal; now it can be treated. Rather, the point is that health care has been shifting more and more to a highly specialized, high-tech emphasis in which the individual's needs and the prevention of disease have taken a backseat to expensive hospitals and superspecialized physicians.

Fortunately, we do not have to decide if we were better off then or now. There are ways that we can take advantage of the best of both worlds. We can have high-tech interventions in those cases in which it really is necessary and valuable, and we can have an emphasis on producing a healthy population that mostly does not need such expensive interventions. But change necessitates a new understanding of how the individual fits into the health environment.

The most important questions in modern health care should not be focused around artificial hearts and cancer chemotherapy but rather around the question "Who stays well?" Surprisingly, there is good evidence that it is possible to have fewer physicians, fewer hospitals, and a healthier population.

Sometime before the end of the century, a U.S. government—appointed commission will conclude that certain improvements to the mental health of the general population will produce physically healthier and more productive workers, reducing health care costs. The surgeon general will issue a report. Unfortunately, this probably will occur later rather than sooner. It takes a long time before the knowledge of a few scientists makes its way into the mainstream of public consciousness. For instance, many scientists knew of the dangers of cigarette smoking years before public policy was affected. But perhaps this time we will be lucky and the tremendous pressures to save health care dollars will result in quicker action.

MIRACULOUS RESULTS WITHOUT MIRACLES

In short, this book tells the story of the relationship between personality and health as revealed by the latest scientific evidence. It describes the links between personality and disease, and it looks at personalities that stay healthy. In other words, this book presents the first analysis of the *self-healing personality* and its opposite, the disease-prone personality. Finally, this book evaluates the implications for the individual and for health care.

Among the questions addressed are: When is stress harmful and when is it *not* harmful? What is the latest scientific word on the coronary-prone personality? Can hard work protect against, rather than cause, heart disease? Why are meditation and biofeedback not for everyone? Why shouldn't most people worry about eggs in their diet? Is there really a cancer-prone personality? Which psychological techniques of coping with cancer may prolong life? What are the implications for sufferers of arthritis, asthma, diabetes, and migraines? What can be done to improve health without extensive psychotherapy or expensive technological intervention?

This is not a book about miracles. Undoubtedly, there are cases in which people make spectacular recoveries from serious illness through their own force of will, but such cases are uncommon. On the other hand, many millions of people could be helped if the recently unmasked role of psychological factors in health were better understood. When all of the evidence is brought together, an exciting new picture of healing emerges.

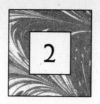

2

How Can Personality Be Related to Health?

Educated people know that simply wishing upon a star or meditating in front of a guru will not cure their cancer. All too often, they and their physicians pooh-pooh the idea that their heart disease, cancer, or arthritis could be influenced by psychological factors. On the other hand, people know that there are certain stressful situations that give them headaches, backaches, nausea, or chest pain. They also recall the beneficial effects of some mental states—times in their lives when they are psychologically exhilarated and become fit as a fiddle. In other words, many people hold contradictory notions about the relationship between psychology and health.

An interesting case revealing the importance of individual personality in achieving health concerns a thirty-five-year-old woman who for about six years was increasingly bothered by a cluster of symptoms in her lower abdominal region. Sara felt bloated before her menstrual period and very "crampy" during her period. She was often constipated and her abdomen ached intermittently, despite an adequate diet. She had pain in her lower back almost every morning. Although miserable and grumpy, she was always able to continue her work as an advertising executive.

Because Sara's symptoms might have been caused by a number of serious medical conditions, she underwent several series of X rays—expensive, unpleasant, and even potentially dangerous. But these and all other medical tests were negative. The normal test results plus the fact that Sara's general health remained good led her gynecologist and her family practitioner to conclude that Sara's problems were "functional." (This, in essence, means that no known drug or surgical intervention would likely effect a cure.) They suggested that perhaps she was under too much stress. Her gynecologist told her that introverted, sensitive women like Sara were prone to cramping, but no one knew why. Her family practitioner recommended that she lose some weight and take up jogging.

Sara did stop eating desserts, and she occasionally went jogging. But she felt funny running around in a jogging suit, and besides, she said, "How can I go jogging when I have a full-time job, my choir practice, and a new romantic relationship that I'm trying to deal with?"

At work soon afterward, Sara was having one of her "bad days," and her boss introduced her to a young, hot-shot gynecologist who was opening a chain of premenstrual syndrome (PMS) clinics. Over lunch she mentioned her symptoms, and he quickly exclaimed, "I can fix you up." After reviewing Sara's past test results and doing a thorough exam, he prescribed a promising new drug that disturbs usual hormonal patterns. Unfortunately, Sara had a severe reaction to the drug and immediately had to cease taking it.

The one good result of the intense drug reaction was that it scared Sara into making an appointment with the head of the gynecology department at a large university medical center. This doctor had treated a thousand Saras. He looked over Sara's medical history and talked to her in his office for forty-five minutes, then asked her to go to the examining room for an exam.

During their next visit, the doctor looked Sara in the eye and announced, "I'm going to be able to help you." Together they worked out a comprehensive program of special exercises, temporary medication, changes in diet, and extensive but gradual changes in her work and relaxation habits—a systematic program that incorporated help from her boyfriend and her girlfriends. All of the changes were tailored to Sara's particular background, bodily reactions, habits, and personal situation. Four months later, Sara was well on her way to recovery.

No one—except for Sara—was particularly surprised when Sara

finally overcame her health problems. Those who knew her recognized that Sara's new life-style was a far better match for her personality. She seemed so much more content and serene, and she was even more enthusiastic and creative in her work. Yet no one had been able to help her during those six years of suffering.

Many people are strangely resistant to the idea that they should actively work on their psychological makeup in order to improve their physical condition. The same physicians who advise their patients to "take it easy" are unlikely to add intensive "personality treatment" to the usual regimen of drugs, exercise, and dietary control assigned to people at high risk for a heart attack.

Why this general unwillingness to relate personality—the individual's persistent patterns of responding to life's challenges—to serious illness? Part of the reason is that most people and most physicians are made skeptical by far-out miracle cures constantly promoted by hucksters of all sorts. And part of the reason is that true psychological influences are gradual and undramatic; they lack the sense of theater of major surgery or wonder drugs.

Another reason personality is often ignored in health care is that people are used to thinking of the mind as separate from the body. Mental matters are the province of psychologists and psychiatrists, not cardiologists and oncologists. This separation, or dualism, narrows the thinking of health care professionals.

But the main reason personality is too often ignored is that a psychological and social, or *psychosocial*, approach does not fit into the traditional mechanical approach to illness.

Automobile mechanics do not insure that the roads are smooth, that the gasoline is high quality, and that the drivers are well trained. They simply fix the car when something breaks or deteriorates. Analogously, the health care system generally is not designed to promote the individual's health. Physicians mainly fix things that go wrong; through no fault of their own, they do not do much about keeping people healthy. They know an awful lot about anatomy, biochemistry, and pharmacology, but not much about psychology, family relations, or nutrition. I was surprised when I studied a pediatric residency program (postgraduate medical training for pediatricians) and found that many pediatricians learn very little if anything about normal psychological development.

This extreme technical orientation also is reflected in and perpetuated by the economic reward system in health care. Not long ago, I talked to the director of one of the world's leading training programs for cardiologists. This distinguished woman asked and then answered an important question: "What do I get paid for an hour of my time? I get paid the *least* for an hour spent talking to and evaluating a new patient, the place where my abilities and experience are probably *most* valuable and *most* needed."

Which medical procedures cost the most, and which physicians get paid the most? An ophthalmologist who uses a laser to reattach the retina in an injured eye may earn a small fortune in just a few years. (And, of course, it is wonderful that such a medical procedure exists.) Likewise, a surgeon who removes a gall bladder and relieves the patient of excruciating pain would be well compensated.

A pediatrician who spends an hour convincing a fourteen-year-old to stay off cocaine or tobacco earns, after deducting overhead expenses, about enough to buy a chef's salad for lunch at the local diner. Despite some recent efforts to correct these economic imbalances, the problem remains. A home health care attendant, nurse, or social worker who spends every day keeping a group of frail elderly persons at home well nourished, happy, and away from expensive nursing homes, probably does not earn enough money to support a family. Health promotion and the psychological and behavioral aspects of health care are poorly attended to and undercompensated.

The ancient Greeks did not understand physiology, but they did understand the importance of internal harmony and a proper psychosocial atmosphere. However, the ancient Greeks' attention to maintaining health through internal balance, dominant in medicine for many centuries, has all but disappeared in today's high-tech, fix-it health care system. Surprisingly, though, it is science, not humanism, that will correct this sad state of affairs.

ALL BODIES ARE NOT EQUAL

Most people do not react to any given situation just as their friends react. We all have different personalities, different emotional reaction patterns, and different illnesses. In a group of three women I know, one develops rashes when she is nervous, another gets headaches, and the third diarrhea.

The causes of nervousness differ, too. Some people hate getting up in front of an audience, some go crazy sitting at a desk all day, and others dread travel, dogs, sex, exams, or the boss. And most people know these things about themselves. Sir Francis Bacon, in the year 1625, put it this way: "A man's own observation, what he finds good of and what he finds hurt of, is the best physic to preserve health."

Some of these individual differences are genetically based. Just as bodies come in different shapes, sizes, and colors, they also come with different metabolisms, nervous systems, and internal organs. Other individual differences arise from the environments in which we live—the family environment, the social environment, the nation, the culture. Although these assertions sound perfectly reasonable and obvious when stated in this way, they are almost totally ignored in health care.

In the 1950s, the psychiatrist Stewart Wolf described a case of what he called "hyperemesis gravidarum praecox." Translated from the ridiculous jargon so often used in medical care, this phrase means that the female patient vomited at the mention of pregnancy. It is, of course, well known that many women feel nauseous early in pregnancy, as their hormonal balance shifts. But this poor woman vomited even at the *thought* of pregnancy. Her hormones shifted as she talked about pregnancy. The point is that the internal environment is affected by the external environment, but in different ways for different people.

I like to write in the morning. I find that I can be most clear and creative at that time. In an interview several years ago, Bob Hope reported using the morning for things that need little creativity or concentration. He said he was more alert later in the day. Does this mean that one of us is wrong? Obviously not. Does this mean that only Bob Hope's followers can live a long life? I hope not. It is not surprising that different people have different daily rhythms. People have different bodies. What is surprising is that our health care system does very little to take these differences into account.

A number of years ago, sociologist Mark Zborowski showed marked ethnic differences in response to pain. English Protestants ("Yankees") were inclined to be stoic and to deny pain. Italian patients were more expressive and sought relief from the pain. Jewish patients also reacted in an emotional manner, but they tended to be more concerned with the cause of the pain and its significance for the future. Wouldn't it make sense to consider these differences to be an important aspect of health?

In Australia there is a computer-related health epidemic called "repetitive strain injury." Computer operators, most commonly women working in offices, develop all sorts of pains in their fingers, hands, and arms. It is a major source of medical costs and missed work. Yet this health problem is almost unknown in the United States and other industrialized countries that use the same computers. Something about the Australian culture, not anything biological, encourages this serious health problem. Relatedly, Americans are very likely to seek and receive drugs and surgery from their doctors, while the British are likely to receive far more conservative treatment. The French are likely to use unproven nutritional and drug treatments that are not used or are outlawed by the Food and Drug Administration (FDA) in the United States. Yet Americans, the British, and the French are about equally healthy overall.

In Japan there are well-defined social expectations. Many of these norms concern cooperation with the group and polite deference toward others' feelings. A Japanese individual who is loud-mouthed, aggressive, and brusque will face sanctions by the society and probably will feel distressed as a result. He or she may be labeled "sick" or "crazy." In the United States or Italy or Israel, the opposite is common. It is the shy, reserved, and deferent individual who is likely to feel unsuccessful and isolated. *The mismatch between person and society can be a main source of stress and an important factor in illness.*

How can we possibly measure individual differences and know a person's health needs? One way is through the use of psychosocial screening measures as supplements to the traditional biological testing. We can determine an individual's psychological predisposition (for example, shy or outgoing), social environment (for example, a large family), job demands (for example, high status, long hours), and so on. We can then observe the person's resulting emotional style.

Another simple and informative assessment approach is to ask the individual directly. Many people know their own psychological strengths and weaknesses. For example, one of the "discoveries" of researchers studying relapse among people addicted to cigarettes and other harmful substances is that the best predictor of relapse is the question: "Do you think you have kicked the habit, or do you think you may have a relapse?"

Yet this is rarely done. For example, take the case of a pregnant woman. Pregnancy and the postnatal period are high-risk times. Internal hormones fluctuate dramatically, and as people react to the woman's new status, external social influences can be equally dramatic. Some women react to the pressures by becoming depressed, angry, or otherwise upset; they then may smoke, drink, take drugs, eat poorly, miss sleep, and so on, all very dangerous things for both mother and baby. Yet obstetricians will perform all sorts of high-tech tests on the fetus and the newborn but will almost never do a detailed psychological assessment of the mother. And even the best, most sensitive obstetrician is unlikely to ever have an in-depth, personal discussion with the baby's father. It is simply not part of the physician's training and expertise.

In short, there are tremendous individual differences in adults' psychological makeup that should be, but rarely are, taken fully into account in maintaining health. Basically these differences revolve around emotional imbalances; this issue is the theme of this book.

RESPONSIBILITY FOR HEALTH

Not that long ago, a major corporation tried to limit the health insurance benefits available to its employees. The company said it would deny benefits for illness caused by certain "life-style" factors. For example, if you went to a prostitute and contracted AIDS, or if you abused drugs and became sick, you would not be covered by insurance. In this way, the company could control costs and thus provide good coverage for its other employees.

Of course, there was a tremendous uproar. Aside from the practical difficulties of implementing such a plan, many people thought it was cruel and unfair. In general, people are very uncomfortable with the idea that they play some important role in maintaining their own health. We know that any of us can get sick, and it is not necessarily our fault.

Life insurance companies have long denied benefits for policyholders who commit suicide. Yet it would seem unfair to withhold benefits from a lung cancer patient who still is smoking cigarettes. This ambivalence is due to several factors. First, although we generally believe we have some control over our lives, we also know that some aspects of what we do are beyond our control. We did not pick our genes and we cannot always control our environment; we may be "hooked" on cigarettes. Second, we all make mistakes sometimes, so it does not seem fair to penalize a neighbor who made a mistake that led to an illness. Third, we know that to some extent illness is the result of bad luck, so we hesitate to assign blame.

Although there is no benefit in blaming ourselves for our illnesses, the other side of the coin is that we often hesitate to take responsibility for our health. We are so used to assuming that health and disease are a function of fate or of societal influences beyond our control that we do not worry about our health until we get sick. Even at that point, we often turn over responsibility to our physicians. However, the more I learn about personal and emotional factors in health, the more I become convinced that our health can be vastly improved. But the existing health care system will not do it for us. We have to do much of it ourselves.

Some readers of this book will see it as an indictment of physicians and other health care professionals, but such a view is incorrect. Most doctors are dedicated, hard-working, and well-trained professionals who do what they are trained to do. They are among the most productive members of our society. The problem lies with our overall health care system, a system in which we have placed physicians, disease, drugs, and technology at the center and shunted disease resistance, health promotion, social and emotional health, public health, and inner healing off to the fringes. Once this emphasis changes, it will be perfectly obvious that personality is related to health.

A self-healing personality is, in part, a personality that lives a life appropriate for that person. An appropriate view of health takes into account that people are more than machines, and it understands that there are marked differences among individuals. And, finally, it understands that people ultimately have some responsibility for their own health. Most people, upon reflection, know (or can learn) which things are good or bad for them, but rarely are they encouraged to consider psychosocial influences on their well-being or to take primary responsibility for their own health.

It is not the case that most modern-day morbidity and mortality are caused by exotic infections, worn-out organs, or striking genetic defects that demand the attention of superspecialized physicians. Rather, human emotions and human behaviors are central. The diseases of our times are those slow-developing and chronic conditions that involve a wide range of bodily systems.

If personality is indeed so relevant to health, then the potential to improve health and reduce suffering is phenomenal. But exactly how does personality affect health? There is more than one answer to this question.

PATHS LINKING PERSONALITY AND HEALTH

Some newborns are quiet and sleep a lot. Others are active and alert. Similarly, some babies are calm, while others are irritable. When a two-month-old infant screams incessantly, the pediatrician tells the anxious parents that the baby has colic. This label just means that the baby is irritable and screams a lot; nobody really knows why.

Anyone who works in a nursery knows that some babies are inhibited and fearful and some are more outgoing and extroverted. They are born with a certain genetic temperament or constitution. This powerful influence of genetics has been verified by careful studies that compare infants, that follow children's moods over time, and that investigate twins. These stable individual differences persist throughout childhood and to some extent on into adulthood.

Oskar and Jack are identical twins who did not get to know each other until they were adults. They took part in a research study that lends interesting support to the idea of biological temperament. Like others in the study, these twins have exactly the same set of genes. But due to adoption or other forced separation at birth, they found themselves raised in different social environments. Oskar was raised in Germany by his Catholic maternal grandmother; Jack was raised in Israel by his Jewish father. Psychologists tracked them down and brought them together later in life. It turns out that these brothers share a number of traits, such as absentmindedness and, most important, the same sort of angry temperament. Each of us is born with certain temperamental predispositions.

On the other hand, there is no doubt that personality is greatly influenced by family and environment. A shy, introverted child can become more friendly and outgoing if he or she grows up in an environment that encourages and rewards extroverted behavior. (Changes also can occur in adults—for example, some people have undergone dramatic personality changes after a religious conversion. But this is rare.) In other words, although personality depends partly on biological temperament, it is also heavily shaped by the social environment. Personality is a synthesis of biological tendencies, family upbringing, and the culture and subcultures in which we develop.

The links between underlying biological temperament and health are important because of their implications for encouraging a self-healing personality. Consider the case of Irv, an older man with an aggressive, active, dominant temperament. Attempts by this man's family and doctors to encourage him to become a relaxed, easygoing dawdler failed repeatedly. His genetic predispositions could not be eliminated. On the other hand, attempts to improve Irv's health by channeling his aggressive tendencies in a positive direction were more successful. He learned to be a successful, well-regarded fund-raiser for his alma mater. Emotional balance still could be restored. Changes in adult personality produce more beneficial effects on health if underlying genetic tendencies are taken into account.

In 1947 and 1948, a number of medical students at Johns Hopkins University were studied in terms of their genetic and psychological characteristics. The students were categorized as either slow and solid (wary, self-reliant), rapid and facile (cool, clever), or irregular and uneven (moody, demanding). Then they were followed for thirty years. During that time, about half of the group developed some serious health problem. Most (77 percent) of the previously labeled irregular and uneven types developed some serious disorder during those thirty years, but only about a quarter of the rest had major health problems. In a follow-up study on later classes of Johns Hopkins medical students, the irregular and uneven temperament types were again much more likely to have developed serious health problems or to have died. They seemed constitutionally predisposed to do so.

In sum, one of the paths linking personality and health is through underlying genetic temperament. However, there are also ways in which personality plays a direct role in health. The two main pathways involve an internal physiological route and an external behavioral route.

Stress Links: The Internal Route

Much of the research on stress and health has been conducted on laboratory animals; members of the same genetic strain (such as specially bred mice) can be studied. Holding the genetic strain constant eliminates an important source of unpredictability. (This is not possible in studies of humans, except for those involving identical twins.) Furthermore, rodents have a short life span; it may take decades to detect effects in humans that can been seen in months in rats.

What happens when a rodent is stressed? Mice and rats are likely to develop hypertension (high blood pressure) in a stressful environment. It also has been shown that certain laboratory animals are more likely to develop clogged arteries under stressful conditions than under nonstressful ones, and that certain stresses can cause heart attacks.

Can we generalize these findings and apply them directly to people? Of course not. That is why the links between psychosocial factors and disease have not been absolutely proven. Are there analogies to human health and disease? Without a doubt there are, and the links among stress, emotional reactions, and health are far better established than most people realize.

Consider the case of coronary heart disease, in which fatty plaque builds up in the arteries until the heart loses its supply of blood. If you examine a person who is experiencing high stress, you will find a fast-beating heart and elevated blood pressure. These bodily changes can do direct damage to the artery walls, thus encouraging plaque buildup. Furthermore, if you measure the person's blood, you will find excessive levels of the stress hormones, which can interfere with normal chemical reactions in the blood, thus further encouraging the buildup of plaque.

Next, consider the cases of cancer and arthritis, diseases that often are related to problems involving the immune system. Cancer, arthritis, and many other diseases result in part from defects in the bodily system that protects us from invading microbes and other foreign substances. As we shall see, the immune system is weakened by excessive stress. But the effects—and the disease—are more likely to occur in some people than in others.

Julius Caesar thought that a sudden death was the best kind of death, but I think it depends on one's age and circumstance. The links between stress and disease are sometimes sudden. For example, there is increasing evidence that stress is a causal factor in cardiac arrhythmias—the uncontrolled quivering of the heart that can result in sudden death. Unfortunately, we do not yet have absolute proof of this relationship, because stress-induced arrhythmias usually either cure themselves before the patient can be examined or kill the patient, thereby ending the arrhythmia. When the Hmongs (from Laos) were relocated to the United States in the late 1970s, a shocking number of young, healthy immigrants in their thirties died suddenly in their sleep. The stress of cultural dislocation can be an important element in cases of sudden death.

Here, too, individual differences are important. Significant work in this area has been done by Dr. Bernard Lown and his associates at Harvard. Lown reports on various studies demonstrating the increased likelihood of sudden cardiac death after such stresses as bereavement, unemployment, and even returning to work on Monday morning. But perhaps Dr. Lown's greatest insight recently is his focus on the emotional reactions of the individual.

Lown has found that the most potent stress relates to the recall of an emotionally charged experience. Such psychological stress is uniquely individual. For example, one woman did not develop an arrhythmia (technically a ventricular premature beat, or VPB) when told that she had advanced malignancy (cancer), but she *did* show a cardiac arrhythmia when asked to discuss her homosexual son.

Why do only some people drop dead from emotional shock? Dr. Lown proposes a three-part model to account for the variability in sudden cardiac death after encountering stress. First, some electrical instability must be present already in the heart muscle; this often is due to partially blocked arteries. Second, the person must be feeling a pervasive emotional state such as depression. Third, there must be a triggering event, such as the loss of one's job or the death of a loved one. In this book, we shall delve most deeply into the second of these factors—the harmful effects of an emotional disturbance and the protective effects of a self-healing personality. (Note that there are about 300,000 sudden cardiac deaths in the United States each year, and hundreds of thousands more worldwide.)

In short, a major link between personality and health involves those physiological changes occurring inside our bodies during stress. Although the psychophysiological mechanisms are complex, there is no doubt that they exist and that they are important.

Behavioral Links: The External Route

The other major link between personality and health is behavior. This connection is not so simple as it first sounds.

Any one of us could be hit by lightning or lose a loved one or be involved in an auto accident. Sometimes we just have bad luck. Because such events are seemingly random, we often assume that there is little we can do to protect ourselves. But consider this: Who is more likely to wander aimlessly across a busy street, a happy, fulfilled person or a lonely, depressed, preoccupied person? Who is more likely to go out for a late-night drive alone and without wearing a seat belt? Who is more likely to inject illegal drugs into his or her veins? It is obvious that people who are depressed, lonely, angry, or otherwise psychologically disturbed are more likely to put themselves into unhealthy situations. In other words, one way that personality affects health is through behaviors that lead to more or less healthy habits and environments.

Some people are predisposed to addiction. It is hard to know for sure the extent to which this is determined by genetic temperament or by upbringing (probably both are involved), but there is good evidence that there is an addictive personality. Some people are just more likely than others to overeat, drink too much, get hooked on cigarettes, and so on. In the wrong environment, those with an addictive personality are likely to wind up ruining their health, unless their emotional problems are addressed. In fact, the most important external route through which personality affects health involves our daily habits. Personality problems often lead to unhealthy habits, which in turn help maintain the personality problems while ruining one's health.

In 1935, Dr. Leon Saul described the case of a man with a severe pain in his right testicle. No organic cause could be found. However, in psychoanalysis, the man began relating sexy nighttime dreams. He then realized that every time he woke up at night, he had an erection. As his emotional problems were resolved and his sexual fantasies weakened, the pain in his testicle disappeared. It had merely been the result of prolonged erections.

Similar cases include sore or broken teeth, muscle-tension headaches, flatulence, and skin rashes. Many anxious people grind their teeth during sleep and wake up with sore teeth or aching jaws. Many tense or angry people contract the muscles in the neck (as one might do in response to a cold wind) and thus produce severe headaches. Other people with emotional disturbances swallow excessive air when they speak; the air has nowhere to go except out the other end. And many anxious people overreact to dry skin or a minor itch, scratching it until there is a serious skin rash or even a nerve problem. In all of these cases, personality is a cause of the health problem, but the intervening agency involves our own direct mistreatment of our bodies.

In sum, the final link between personality and health is the external, or behavioral, route. Although this book focuses more on the internal route, the external route is an important one that often works in concert with the direct physiological effects of stress.

Misleading Links

In a magician's illusion, some crucial fact or piece of information is hidden from the audience, and magic seems to occur. Once the missing fact is revealed, the trick appears quite boring and pedestrian. Scientists can fall into similar traps. Sometimes it seems as if personality is affecting health when that is not really the case at all. For example, some researchers of the nature of personality have found that even when they are not more ill, neurotics—people who are anxious or depressed—are more likely to report symptoms and feel sick than are other people. For example, patients with angina (chest pain) do not always have seriously clogged arteries. Anxiety increases one's feelings of pain, and neurotic people may pay more attention to their bodily symptoms. Thus, while it sometimes appears that neurotics are more likely to have disease, the difference is inflated by the fact that they are more likely to *report* feeling ill.

There are other ways that scientists can be misled. Some of them have to do with the samples of patients that are studied. Others have to do with how the data are obtained. For example, if patients with disease are asked about their emotions and are found to be distressed, it may be that the disease caused the distress, not that the distress caused the disease.

There is a story about an employer who tried to see if his employees would work harder in order to make more money or if paying them more money would make them work harder. He instituted a bonus system based on productivity and found that the employees worked harder. Then he raised everyone's pay and found that they worked harder still. The employees worked harder in order to receive more pay *and* because they received more pay. The employer had erroneously assumed that there was only one cause.

Some people are tempted to make a similar mistake regarding the relationship between personality disruptions and health. It does seem to be the case that there are biases that can produce a misleading link between personality and symptoms of ill health. But it is also the case that certain people with certain emotional disturbances are more likely to become ill. The one does not exclude the other!

IGNORANCE IS NOT ALWAYS BLISS

I sometimes hear colleagues or see newspaper columns belittling the importance of health promotion efforts. It is easy to make fun of proposed changes in people's personalities and life-styles. The speaker or writer may point out that danger lurks everywhere. Airplanes can crash, buildings can collapse, terrorists can attack, artificial chemicals are widespread, and an exciting life is often challenging and stressful. This kind of argument usually concludes, "If you want to live a long and healthy life, then stay home, meditate, eat boiled vegetables and drink boiled water, and do a hundred sit-ups every morning." This is supposed to be funny. But my usual reaction is not laughter but disappointment.

I get upset because this sort of commentary is poorly thought out. The fact is that airplanes usually do *not* crash, buildings usually do not collapse, many tasty and wonderful foods are very healthy for us, and healthy people generally have a more exciting and interesting life than do those who feel ill or are disabled in some way.

These same commentators never would suggest kiddingly that people should freely drink typhoid-contaminated water on an exciting trip to Southeast Asia, or drink and drive, or be promiscuous and not worry about AIDS or venereal disease. Would a responsible speaker add to the above simplistic prescription: "If you want to be healthy, just stay home, eat whole grains, and don't bother with any crack or speed or downers—but watch out, because you may die of boredom"? Of course not, because many high-risk behaviors are condemned by society. Few responsible people would promote or condone drug abuse. But the new ways to promote health, including those discussed in this book, are not yet well understood by society.

Scientists probably deserve some of the blame for people's generally cynical attitude toward promoting health. Hundreds of findings related to health are reported each year, with little attempt to explain broad themes that are emerging and little attention to the *relative risk* of various behaviors. One study reports that coffee drinking raises the risk of heart attack, and the next study contradicts that finding. On the surface it appears that there is no consensus, no truth.

In fact, however, there are many valid recommendations that most people can follow to improve their health. There are also some steps that government should take. Many of these changes involve the self-healing personality; they go well beyond common sense. My desire to explain these consistent findings in comprehensible terms is the reason I wrote this book.

NEITHER NECESSARY NOR SUFFICIENT

Not everyone who is exposed to an infectious disease will contract the disease. For example, many people who are exposed to the flu virus do not get the flu. However, everyone with typhoid fever has been infected by the salmonella typhosa bacterium, and everyone with flu has been infected by a strain of the flu virus. In other words, the infectious microbe is necessary but not sufficient to cause disease.

We already have seen that some physicians, following the traditional mechanical model, may give insufficient attention to the causes of disease, thus overlooking the factors that keep some people healthy. However, there is another important misunderstanding that leads many traditional health providers astray.

I know a man in his sixties who eats fatty foods, smokes cigarettes, is overweight, and never exercises. He is in good health. Why? For unknown reasons, he has beaten the odds. Many people who smoke cigarettes do not get lung cancer, and not everyone with lung cancer has smoked cigarettes. People who eat fatty foods do not automatically develop heart disease, and not everyone with heart disease has eaten a high-fat diet. In other words, for many life-threatening diseases, the risk factors are neither necessary *nor* sufficient causes!

This unsettling state of affairs makes science difficult. In many individual cases, a physician faces a high-risk uncooperative patient who goes merrily on his way, seemingly living forever. Analogously, in many scientific studies, people who are expected to be at higher risk for disease do not turn out to be more likely to develop the disease, because some factors (usually unknown) are unaccounted for. This complex state of affairs is very frustrating for those scientists looking for simple, direct evidence of a personality-to-disease link.

For a number of reasons, personality and stress fall into this category of neither necessary nor sufficient risk factors for disease. Yet, as we shall see, there is excellent evidence that psychosocial factors play a key role in health—that is, that there is a self-healing personality.

Most people know intuitively that the mind should not be separated from the body. Most people know that at certain times in their lives they feel mentally wonderful and physically fit. Their quality of life is improved. But the links between mental status and physical health have not been clearly spelled out for them, especially in terms of their own individual personality.

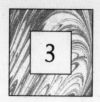

3

Stress: Our Current Understanding

At the turn of the last century, a medical student named Walt Cannon began using the newly discovered X rays to study digestion. He took X rays of the stomach and watched the food pass through. Almost by accident, he noticed that stomach movements seemed to be affected by emotional state. Digestion was not an immutable process; stomach contractions changed as a function of emotional excitement.

As often happens in scientific research, this serendipitous finding had a major impact on scientific thinking. Three decades later, Dr. Walter B. Cannon, by then a famous professor of medicine at Harvard, wrote a fascinating account of how bodily changes occur in association with emotional distress.

Cannon observed that stress causes an increase in the level of sugar in the blood, a large output of adrenaline (epinephrine), an increase in pulse rate and breathing rate, and an increase in the amount of blood pumped to the skeletal muscles. Cannon called this the "fight-or-flight" response. It is well documented in animal studies. When an animal perceives a threatening situation, its reflex response prepares it either for running away or for fighting. This response also can be thought of as one of energy mobilization.

As most people know from personal experience, the inborn fight-

or-flight response exists in stressed humans as well as in threatened animals. It is a product of our evolutionary history. But there are not many saber-toothed tigers walking around my neighborhood. Although there are some dangerous dark alleys, the stresses of today's society usually do not require the fight-or-flight response for actual survival. Yet stressful life events do trigger continuous bodily arousal, and this continuous arousal can cause lasting changes in basic physiological processes. This process is especially likely to occur in the disease-prone personality. On the other hand, some people do not have much of a stress response or do not react badly to the response.

THE BASIC PHYSIOLOGY OF STRESS
(IN SIMPLE, UNSTRESSFUL TERMS)

The same Dr. Cannon, in 1942, wrote about a phenomenon that he called "voodoo death." There are documented examples of people who have received some kind of curse from a witch doctor, have been overcome with fear, and have died within a few days. One tribeswoman ate some fruit that she later learned was spiritually forbidden. Expecting evil spirits to attack her, she literally scared herself to death. Cannon theorized that the continuous stress on the body from severe emotional activation produced this effect.

When this phenomenon was studied in rats by the scientist Curt Richter, some surprising results emerged. Rats were severely stressed by being placed into vats filled with water. Just like the tribeswoman above, many of the overstressed rats did indeed die suddenly, even though they were good swimmers. But autopsies on the rats did not show the kind of physiological stress that Cannon had predicted. Rather, there seemed to be excessive activity involving the *restorative* aspects of the nervous system. Their hearts slowed down and slowed down until they finally stopped. (If the restorative aspects of the nervous system were blocked with a drug, the rats did not suffer this fate.) So the physiology of stress is more complicated than originally thought.

Richter concluded that the rats died because they gave up all hope of surviving. (When other rats were taken in and out of the water, thus maintaining "hope," they kept on swimming while in the vats.) Translating this into terms that the ancient Greeks would have understood, it seemed as if the rats were overcome by the melancholic humor, not the choleric humor that Cannon had expected. It is useful to think about these matters in terms of the Greek humors because it then becomes easier to see what the two mechanisms—fight or flight and hopelessness—have in common, namely an *imbalance in bodily systems*. Dr. Richter spent the rest of his life studying the physiology of internal balance; he lived to the age of ninety-four.

The importance of internal balance, as applied to stress, is again moving to the forefront of scientific thinking. Many people think of stress as a type of pressure that increases and increases until there is a breaking point. But that is a serious misconception. In fact, stress should be thought of as a disruption, a disharmony, a failure of equilibrium.

Stress involves two basic systems of the body—the nervous system and the endocrine, or hormonal, system. These systems are explained in more detail in chapter 7, but a few basic points should be made here. Most important, the nervous system and the endocrine system are the two systems that provide the links between the mind and the body. What we perceive, what we think, and how we cope all set in motion messages from the brain to the rest of the body.

In the case of the nervous system, the message transmission is almost instantaneous. For example, a terrible sight may cause fainting or may send the heart into the uncontrolled fluttering that results in sudden death. The hormonal system, on the other hand, is slower but longer lasting. Hormones released into the blood can travel throughout the body and disrupt all sorts of usual bodily functions. Hormones provide the "rush" we feel when excited or agitated.

These biological systems prepare the body to meet the demands of the external environment while trying to maintain an internal equilibrium. Cannon called this internal regulation, or balance, the "wisdom of the body." However, when our minds cannot cope with our environment, our internal systems go out of whack.

There is a physiological basis for balance. The most relevant part of the nervous system has two separate components—the first speeds things up and mobilizes the body; the second slows things down and restores the body. These are easily noticed in a colleague of mine. When threatened, his eyes widen, his mouth becomes dry, his breathing accelerates, and he looks quite nervous and jittery. As he relaxes, these effects disappear and he often becomes hungry.

The hormonal system, which complements the nervous system, tries to maintain balance through a fluid *feedback loop* to the brain. When hormone levels in the blood get too high, the brain usually signals for a reduction. Too much arousal and excitement *or* too much overcompensation and relaxation may damage body tissues, impair immune system response, or disrupt the biological rhythms necessary to life and health.

Dr. Cannon's discoveries *almost* changed the course of twentieth-century medical practice. Just as his ideas were making their way into medical thinking, antibiotic drugs were being discovered. These miracle drugs were so effective in curing infectious diseases that so-called internal medicine, with its emphasis on biochemistry and drug treatment, became the dominant force in medicine. However, Cannon's discoveries, together with those of the 1980s and 1990s, may change the course of medical practice in the twenty-first century.

THE WISDOM OF THE BODY

A little more than a century ago, physicians began washing their hands and surgeons stopped wiping their scalpels on dirty rags. The germ theory of disease was being developed and successfully tested. At around the same time, modern scientific understanding of the body's internal equilibrium, or *homeostasis*, was begun with the work of Claude Bernard, the great nineteenth-century French physiologist. Despite the influence of the times, Bernard kept his attention not on germs but on the *milieu interne* ("internal environment").

Bernard noted that the key to staying alive and healthy is keeping our cells alive and healthy, and that keeping our cells healthy means maintaining them in an internal environment of a certain temperature, with certain energy (food), with water, with oxygen, with waste disposal, and without toxins or invading, attacking cells. Germs mattered, but often they didn't matter much.

Although the skin does an outstanding job of protecting the body from microorganisms and other threats to health, many microbes do penetrate this first layer of defense. Yet we usually do not become ill.

Various other defenses are in place to protect us. Health is more a dynamic struggle for equilibrium than an absence or avoidance of disease. Furthermore, some people are much better able to maintain this internal equilibrium than are others.

Our immune systems are constantly seeking out and eliminating particles that should not be there, thus maintaining the internal environment. Some cells die; others are created. With the possible exception of the eccentric millionaire Howard Hughes, who lived the later years of his life isolated in a sterile cocoon, our bodies are never germ-free, but still we usually are not ill.

This insight is not well understood. The practice of medicine is pretty much focused on keeping tiny invaders out of our bodies or on killing them once they infect us, not on strengthening our natural resistance to disease. A prominent exception here is the use of vaccines to produce immunity to certain diseases.

GENERALLY SICK

A friend of mine, angry at her doctor, told me that she was thinking about switching physicians. What was the problem? She went to her doctor, complaining "I feel sick." She felt tired and weak and had a headache and loss of appetite, intermittent sleep disturbances, and general aches and pains. (She had no fever, weight loss, or physical impairments.) To a physician, these symptoms are not very interesting in themselves. They are characteristic of many, many illnesses. The physician's job is to find out which illness you have. The main emphasis of medical training is the so-called differential diagnosis. The physician wants to make a specific diagnosis, such as flu, or cancer, or hepatitis, so that proper treatment can be instituted. So her physician tested her blood, urine, and stool, took a chest X ray, and did a physical exam. Everything was normal, and he told her, "You're in good health. Don't worry. Let me know if the symptoms worsen."

The problem with this medical approach is that the general disturbance is immediately overlooked in the search for a specific cause. The fact that the overall bodily upset may be important is ignored.

This problem was first noticed in the 1930s by a young endocrinologist named Hans Selye. Selye was looking for new sex hormones, and so he was injecting cells derived from ovaries into rats to see if their bodies would react. Sure enough, he found an enlargement of the rats' adrenal glands in response to the injections. The adrenal glands are small triangular tissues that sit on top of the kidneys. The adrenal medulla produces such substances as adrenaline. The adrenal cortex produces steroid hormones, such as cortisol (hydrocortisone). Selye, only twenty-eight years old, was ecstatic that he had discovered a new sex hormone that would directly affect a key part of the endocrine system.

Selye's excitement was short-lived, however, for he soon discovered that he could cause the exact same adrenal enlargement by injecting insulin, or by making the rats hot or cold, or by making them exercise heavily, and so on. The adrenal glands, and particularly the adrenal cortex, enlarged whenever the rats' bodies were challenged. Rather than abandon his project in despair, Selye went on to develop the first modern scientific model of a general stress response.

Selye saw that the body's release of hormones was an internal response to external threats. If the threats were too severe, some of the body's organs eventually would fail. Selye's model of an organism facing a challenge, struggling to adapt, and sometimes failing—with the result being disease or death—was called the general adaptation syndrome. Because Selye's syndrome was proposed by a hard-nosed biomedical researcher studying real hormones in real laboratory animals, it had the aura of credibility. It became a sort of rallying cry for modern researchers attempting to overcome the low regard generally afforded to stress topics in traditional medical practice. Selye, who was born in 1907 in Vienna and emigrated to work in the United States and Canada in the 1930s, has been called the "stress pioneer." Actually, though, he was working directly in the tradition of Claude Bernard and Walter Cannon. Selye died in 1982, a minor folk hero.

IF THERE'S NO STRESS, YOU'RE DEAD

Although we all are subject to the fight-or-flight response and the general adaptation syndrome, there are also tremendous individual differences in our responses to stress. When challenged or frightened, some people get an upset stomach, feel nauseous, or wet their pants. Some people get chest pain, back pain, or a headache. Others get cold hands and feel their heart skipping beats. Still others in similar situations seem to have no reaction at all. These responses are related to individual proclivities to disease.

The only way to eliminate all of the challenges to body and mind is to die; there is no stress when you're dead. A key to staying healthy is to keep stress at a manageable level. This must be done in different ways and to different degrees by each individual.

Why do people vary in their responses to challenges? For a number of reasons. First, each person is a unique biological being. Just as some people are tall, muscular, and fit, some people have an "iron stomach," a strong heart, "nerves of steel," and so on. Researchers sometimes speak in terms of individual differences in "reactivity," the extent to which the nervous system responds to stimulation. Hans Selye wrote about the "weakest link"—the part of one's body (heart, kidney, or whatever) that is most likely to be impaired by stress. The weakest link tends to run in families; we are likely to develop the same medical problems faced by our parents and grandparents.

When Selye was a medical student in Prague, he was somewhat of a rebel. While his professors emphasized specific remedies for individual diseases, Selye kept noticing the general syndrome of sickness. He saw the same patients as his professors did, but *he viewed them in a different light*; the difference was one of appraisal and interpretation. This same process of interpretation applies to dealing with stressful challenges. People see and react to the same challenges in various ways. That is, another set of reasons for individual differences in response to challenge involve variations in modes of appraisal and coping. Many psychological techniques for improving health thus involve changes in appraisal and coping.

Differences in response to challenge reflect differences in personality—the stable differences in how people experience and respond to the world. Some people are extroverted, sociable, playful, impulsive, or whatever, while others are introverted, unfriendly, reserved, serious, conscientious, and so on. To take a simple example, a child with a nervous disposition who sees his mother get nauseous whenever there is a family quarrel and who is excused from school whenever he has similar symptoms is likely to grow up with a nervous personality that shows this particular sort of response to stress.

Thus, although biological responses to stress are based on universal biological processes, they vary tremendously as a function of the psychology and physiology—or psychophysiology—of the individual. These psychophysiological responses can be modified, so there are means to create a healing personality. But although stress is affected by our interpretations and personalities, most stress does not originate inside of us. Rather, the social environment affects our level of stress.

Major Life Changes

Many people become ill or die following a significant change in their life. Lyndon Johnson died of a heart attack just after his successor, Richard Nixon, began dismantling Johnson's "Great Society" social welfare programs. In turn, soon after Richard Nixon resigned the presidency in disgrace, he became seriously ill with phlebitis and his wife Patricia had a stroke. On the other hand, three of the first five U.S. presidents—John Adams, Thomas Jefferson, and James Monroe— died on the Fourth of July. Was it because they were able to resist death and keep themselves alive until this special date?

When a person becomes seriously ill soon after the death of a loved one, the old wisdom is that the person is suffering from a "broken heart." In fact, widows and widowers are indeed more likely to die than are those who are not bereaved. But not all widowed people become ill or follow their partners into the grave. The issue is more complicated than that.

Dr. Adolf Meyer, an influential physician who emigrated from Switzerland to the United States at the turn of the century, came to the conclusion that the psychosocial events in a person's life are a prime determinant of illness. He developed a "life chart" to record the detailed psychosocial history of each of his patients. Like Drs. Lown and Selye, Dr. Meyer thought that the meaning (significance) of the events to the individual was most important.

Meyer's efforts were taken up in the 1950s by researchers who developed scales to measure stressful life events. They then used these scales in questionnaires to see whether people with serious illnesses had encountered special stress during the preceding six months to a year. More important, they measured large numbers of people and then followed them to see if stressful life changes produced illness in the year or so that followed.

Drs. Thomas Holmes, Richard Rahe, and colleagues did indeed find an increased likelihood of disease following stressful events. Their research began on young men in the U.S. Navy and involved minor illnesses. But the studies progressed to older people and more serious illnesses. Some of this latter research took place in Sweden and Finland. (Public health researchers like to conduct research in Scandinavia because excellent information is available about the social, economic, and health status of almost everyone in the population.) Those people with significant life stresses were two to three times more likely to experience major health problems, such as heart attacks.

Although efforts at assessing major life changes began over fifty years ago, they still are not a standard aspect of medical care. Many fine physicians will indeed probe deeply into a patient's total life story, but many more choose not to bother. Part of the reason is, of course, that psychosocial events are not part of the traditional medical approach to disease. A second reason these events are ignored is that they often are difficult to interpret—some people do not find it stressful to move five times in five years; others find it very stressful.

Because some individuals seem to do just fine even when facing many changes in their lives, attention has shifted to trying to understand exactly what it is about change that can be harmful. Thus our understanding of stress has become much more sophisticated.

Most of our major life challenges relate to work, school, love, family, money, place of residence, friends, or health. Therefore, in the most simplistic analysis, the most stable, balanced people would be a happily married couple working at the same steady jobs, living in the same, unchanging neighborhood, and with the same network of friends. Although most people cannot remain in such a setting, this stability does turn out to be a very healthy environment. For example, in a dramatic study of a stable, close-knit Italian-American community in Rosetto, Pennsylvania, it was found that heart disease rates were much lower than in nearby, less-stable towns, even though the residents of Rosetto were eating an unhealthy, high-fat diet.

On the other hand, people who relish a lot of stimulation can undergo many life changes without feeling distressed. Some challenges are not harmful to some people. On the contrary, they represent good stress.

STRESS AND THE HEALTHY INDIVIDUAL: GOOD STRESS

If you put an eight-month-old child in a room full of unusual objects, the child probably will not hide his or her head under a blanket. Rather than avoid challenge, the child will strike out and explore.

Many adults choose to tackle maddening puzzles, or engage in competitive sports, or travel to exotic locales. All of these activities are stressful in the sense of being challenging, but often the challenge is not harmful, but stimulating.

In fact, various sorts of evidence suggest that curiosity, stimulation, and exploration are important elements of a healthy individual. People have an innate desire to explore and master their worlds. Many people report feeling most alive when they face a stimulating new job, a new love, or a new home. Selye came to call the agreeable challenges *eustress*, meaning "good stress" (as opposed to "distress"). It has even been shown that boredom is stressful and leads to the release of stress hormones. In one study, monotonous work was a significant correlate of heart disease.

What about moving frail and depressed eighty-year-old Aunt Edna into a hut in the Australian outback so that she can develop a new sense of adventure? I would not recommend it, unless the goal is to see the last of Aunt Edna. The challenges of new tasks and environments become harmful if we are not fit enough to address them, if they are overwhelming, or if we face other emotional problems at the same time.

Almost everyone has a story about a parent, grandparent, or old friend who died soon after being widowed. But when we hear about a person's dying after learning of the death of a loved one, the second victim is almost never a young person. Typically it is the sixty-six-year-old widower, not the twenty-five-year-old war widow, who follows the spouse into death. Stress is most detrimental when the body is already damaged or ill to some extent.

TIMING OF STRESS

The recovery period after an illness or surgery is not the healthiest time to enter a marathon or change jobs. A key factor affecting the impact of stress involves the body's existing state of health.

Even hamsters can develop heart disease. A particular strain of hamsters inherits heart disease that develops in a regular pattern, similar to that of human heart disease. When these hamsters are studied in a controlled laboratory setting, researchers can be confident that any effects of stress are not due to extraneous factors. (People do not always follow the instructions of a scientific experimenter, but hamsters have little choice.) One study went as follows.

On Monday mornings, the hamsters woke up from their restful weekend and "went to work." That is, they were stressed by the researchers. And so it went, Tuesday, Wednesday, Thursday, and Friday. A control group of hamsters was not stressed. Later, the animals were examined for evidence of heart failure. Two important findings emerged. First, only the hamsters who had a hereditary tendency toward heart disease developed heart disease. Second, the effects of the stress were greater on those disease-prone hamsters that already had begun to develop heart disease. In other words, stress had its greatest effects on those who already were weakened.

Hamsters are not people, and no one to my knowledge has studied the hamster personality. However, there is a variety of evidence that healthy, disease-resistant persons can fight off the harmful effects of stress. (The exact nature of the disease-resistant personality is explained in detail in chapter 6.) People who are beginning to develop a disease anyway are likely to be severely impacted by stress.

There are likely other times that stress is more harmful, but these have not been studied much. One interesting line of research, though, looks at the timing of heart attacks in terms of hour of the day. The evidence is fairly clear that people are more likely to suffer a heart attack in the early morning as opposed to, say, late in the afternoon, after a full day's work. The reasons for this are unclear. But people who have their own hunches about the times and seasons that they feel most vulnerable to stress would do well to act to reduce unnecessary challenges at those times.

HASSLES

At Christmastime, the newspapers sometimes run detailed stories about families that are really down on their luck. Here is one from my local paper: The father of the family had a severe heart attack and lost his job. The family could not make the mortgage payments, so they lost their house. They moved to California with the promise of a new job, but it fell through, and they wound up in a shelter for the homeless. Health outcome for this family? As expected, if bad event after bad event assaults you and you have nowhere to turn, health problems are likely; slowly but surely, the health of this family was deteriorating.

Fortunately, most people do not face such a series of catastrophes. Instead, our stress usually seems to come from an overwhelming series of minor events, such as being yelled at by the boss, being cheated by a salesman, and being stuck every day in heavy traffic. Intuitively we know that such daily hassles can cause pains in our necks or make us feel stressed. Can the cumulative effect of daily hassles become serious? Analogously, could minor daily uplifts, such as a walk in the park or a good joke, reduce stress and improve health?

In one interesting study of well-educated adults in the San Francisco area, the frequency and intensity of daily hassles was significantly related to degree of illness. In another study of elderly persons with osteoarthritis, hassles again were related to self-reported physical health over a six-month period. To get a sense of these hassles, you might try the following exercise: For one week, carry around a small notebook and make a brief note whenever you do such things as misplace your car keys, face a home maintenance chore, run short of money, worry about a family member, have too many things to do, and so on. Then compare your feelings of stress and health to those of another week, when you encounter fewer hassles. The difference is usually quite dramatic.

The physiological basis for these effects is starting to become clear.

An overwhelming series of hassles can produce a chronically negative mood. And fluctuations in mood are related to blood pressure, metabolism, and the strength of the immune system. For example, a person's immune system response (antibody response) will be lower on days when he or she has a relatively high degree of negative moods.

THE RIGHT PERSON
IN THE WRONG ENVIRONMENT
(AND VICE VERSA)

I enjoy swimming and, living in San Diego, I can swim most days. Not too long ago, I was paddling along when I was joined and passed by a woman furiously doing the crawl stroke. When she stopped briefly to catch her breath, she muttered to me, "Now I know why I quit this years ago." I looked puzzled and simply asked, "Why?" She responded, "Because I hate it."

This woman was not overweight, so she was not swimming because of a need to burn off excess calories. She was swimming because someone told her that exercise was good for her. She did not ask me for my opinion, so I did not offer any advice. But my guess is that she was doing her body more harm than good through this fine aerobic exercise. She hated the task and she hated the pressures; judging from her clenched teeth and angry face, it is likely that harmful stress hormones were flowing.

Oftentimes the source of stress can be found neither in the person nor in the person's environment. Instead the problem lies in the match, or actually with the *mis*match, between the person and the environment. Stress results when our thoughts and feelings conflict with the demands of the situation.

Is there any proof of the common assertion that job stress is unhealthy? Some of the best evidence on this question has been provided by Dr. Joseph E. Schwartz and his colleagues. Dr. Schwartz is a mellow fellow himself, and his job as a medical school professor allows him plenty of flexibility in allocating his time. But what about an assembler who wants to have some say in his work but is denied by the factory management? Is this conflict between the worker's desires and the demands of the job stressful and damaging to health?

It is not easy to find good data to answer this question. Few studies gather job information and health status from large groups of people. But Dr. Schwartz figured out a way to estimate job characteristics based on some large-scale census studies. The researchers, led by Dr. Robert Karasek, then defined job strain in terms of psychological demands and decision latitude. Psychological demands included things like having to work too hard and fast and facing conflicting demands. Decision latitude included having a lot of say on the job, having variety in the work, and having jobs that require creativity.

In a high-strain job, there are many demands but little decision latitude. High-strain jobs include assemblers, cooks, waiters, cashiers, and office computer operators. Low-strain jobs generally include foresters, salespeople, architects, and repairmen.

The research of Karasek and Schwartz showed that high job strain people were more likely to suffer heart attacks. This remained true even after traditional risk factors (such as age and blood pressure) were taken into account. Why? Another study, at a Swedish sawmill where workers faced repetitive, high-speed tasks over which they had no control, found that this high-strain work led to high levels of stress hormones being released by the workers' bodies.

Sociologists have demonstrated that jobs that are disturbing and uncontrollable are the most harmful. They involve a sense of psychological impotence—a feeling that, at least for a while, the person is totally unable to cope with the changes in the environment. In the extreme, the person loses self-esteem and interest in life and in other people. As we shall see, this sense of hopelessness is one key aspect of the disease-prone personality.

Although very informative, what these studies are missing is the person's own perspective. That is, they do not study the individual in depth to see how he or she feels about the job situation. If they did, I believe they would find that some people are perfectly content with being told exactly what to do, whereas others feel out of place and conflicted, the latter group being even more likely to develop health problems than has previously been imagined.

In general, the recent refinements in our understanding of stress point to the importance of the individual. A series of negative life events will be challenging to most people, but many will *not* become ill. People have different biological material to start with, and individuals differ in how they appraise, interpret, and cope with changes. But perhaps most central is one's pattern of emotional responding. People who have chronically negative patterns of emotional responding to challenge also have associated pathological physiologies. But those who respond with a balanced and self-appropriate pattern are far more likely to maintain or regain their health.

Negative Emotions
and Health

In a broad sense, the idea that stress is harmful to health is almost a truism. The real challenge is to explain the stress-to-health link in precise and proven terms. The claim of this book is that it is not stressful environments per se but rather the chronic negative emotions that result from placing certain people into certain environments that is a contributor to much illness. When the relationships between diseases and these negative emotional patterns are examined, the clarity of the associations is striking. Initial reports of these associations sent shock waves through the scientific community as researchers scrambled to reevaluate their thoughts on stress and disease.

In the next chapter, my examinations of disease-prone personalities are presented in detail. First, an analysis is needed of the relevant emotional aspects of personality, especially including the nonverbal emotional styles that are tip-offs that something is awry. It was my experiences in researching nonverbal emotional styles that led to my discoveries regarding the self-healing personality.

NEUROTICISM AND ANXIETY

In common parlance, practically anyone with just about any hang-up may be called "neurotic." It is interesting that the term *neurosis*, meaning a "disorder of the nervous system," came about well before anyone knew that the nervous system really was the key element in being neurotic. But it is important to be clear about what we mean in a technical sense. When accurately used, the term *neuroticism* refers not to a state of craziness but to an emotional disturbance. Neurotic people feel anxious and upset but do not have hallucinations or other problems with understanding reality.

People high on the personality dimension of neuroticism are emotionally unstable, worrying, high-strung, insecure, and vulnerable. On the other hand, people low in neuroticism are calm, at ease, secure, relaxed. Another way to think about neuroticism is in terms of a general propensity toward negative feelings, especially anxiety and sudden anger.

In the biblical Proverbs (chapter 15) is the saying "Better a dinner of vegetables with love than a well-fattened ox with hatred." (Of course, today we also may question the wisdom of eating a fatty ox, but the point of the proverb remains well taken.) The sentiment is echoed in *Aesop's Fables* ("The Town Mouse and the Country Mouse"): "A crust eaten in peace is better than a banquet partaken in anxiety."

Anxiety involves tension and apprehension. Anxiety appears when one senses that something threatening and unpredictable may occur. For example, most people feel some anxiety when caught in the middle of a thunderstorm. Anxiety is closely related to fear, and it also may have elements of guilt and excitement.

Although anxiety is an emotional state that involves physiological arousal, some anxiety is healthy. It is part of the general and universal fight-or-flight pattern. Anxiety becomes a problem only for someone who experiences it in response to a wide variety of situations. Such a person is physiologically anxiety-prone, not simply anxious.

Why is some anxiety healthy? Because it indicates an awareness of and an interest in one's environment. It is only natural and healthy to experience some anxiety before acting in a play ("stage fright") or taking an exam ("test anxiety") or getting married ("having cold feet"). Such anxiety indicates that one is actively addressing and embracing challenge. It is only chronic anxiety that disrupts our basic systems of emotional responding and upsets the body's equilibrium. Chronic anxiety often is associated with depression.

When anxiety becomes a dominant element that interferes with a person's daily functioning, the clinical diagnosis of "anxiety disorder" is applied. Examples include people who are phobic (pathologically fearful) of snakes, of riding in elevators, or even of going outside their homes. Some people who have experienced a terrible event, such as a rape or a bloody battlefield, suffer from frequent, severe anxiety attacks; this is termed "post-traumatic stress disorder." Of course, people with extreme anxiety disorders have a lot of problems in addition to those with their health.

My research shows that anxiety is associated with almost all illness, but common anxiety, though unpleasant, is usually not a threat to health by itself. Anxious people may worry more about their health than others do, and they may be more sensitive to pain. But it is usually only when negative feelings develop into a more severe emotional disturbance, such as a phobia, chronic hostility, depression, or emotional suppression and apathy, that health is directly affected.

WHAT IS HOSTILITY?

Most people understand intuitively that anger is closely related to frustration. When Samuel, a forty-five-year-old middle-level manager, learned he would not achieve his desired goal of heading his company's marketing division, he felt tense, hot, and energized. His lips were tight, his brows drawn down and in, and his anger was clearly noticed by others.

Samuel was more than angry, however; he was hostile. Hostility includes anger, but goes a lot further. Hostile people have a predisposition or orientation toward injuring others, whether physically or verbally. Everyone feels momentary flashes of anger, but not everyone carries around a bitterness, or choler. It is this chronic hostility, rather than simple flashes of anger, that is a threat to health.

At their best, hostile people are simply grouchy. At their worst, they are consumed by hatred. As with other emotional predispositions, aspects of hostility are genetically based. This is most easily seen in the very successful efforts to breed aggressive dogs, chickens, or bulls. However, this predisposition must be brought out by chronically frustrating or challenging situations. Even the most vicious dog may behave like a pussycat when at home with its owner.

Benjamin Franklin, who uncovered many secrets to a long, successful life, warned readers to avoid associating with cholerics and their pessimistic, quarrelsome view of life. Hostile, choleric people are easy to spot. They have emphatic gestures and loud voices. They are dominant and forceful. Their lips are tense and their postures are stiff. Cholerics are easily excited and easily frustrated. They may move around a lot and respond aggressively when challenged. In Samuel's case, he fought like a tiger when anyone disagreed with his judgment. So far, Samuel suffers only from headaches, but it would not be surprising to hear that he has collapsed from a heart attack, just as his choleric father did.

Aggressive, hostile people generally are found to have higher levels of the hormone norepinephrine (noradrenaline) in their blood. But it is an oversimplification to say that this hormone is the physiological component of hostility. Rather, since norepinephrine is secreted as a function of various stresses, it more useful to think of it as simply a sign of internal imbalance. As we shall see, this hormone and related physiological reactions play a key role in cardiovascular disease and general disease proneness.

Hostility, of course, has direct implications for our relations with other people. Choleric people are not trusting, helpful, or forgiving. Thus, the consequences of hostility depend to a large extent on the social network in which the hostile person lives.

WHAT IS APATHY?

The glib answer to "What is apathy" is "I don't care"—a funny, perhaps, but faulty answer. Apathy is more accurately defined as the absence or suppression of passion or emotion. What is apathy? "I don't feel." This cool, sluggish style is what the ancient Greeks called "phlegmatic."

A few years ago, fifty healthy college students were brought into a laboratory each day for four consecutive days. All wrote papers, but not the same type of papers. Half of the students were asked to write about the most traumatic and upsetting experiences of their entire lives. The remainder of the students were instructed to write about trivial topics, such as the type of shoes they were wearing. Before and after the writing, blood was drawn from each student and was checked for the power of the immune response. It was found that the students who had written about their traumatic experiences had stronger immune system activity as a result, and they also were less likely to become ill during the following six weeks. This was especially true for those students who previously had held back from discussing the traumatic events.

The unconscious pushing back of threatening feelings from conscious thought usually is termed "repression." When we consciously decide to push back and avoid painful feelings, it is called "suppression." The phlegmatic usually uses both processes, and they both can damage health.

The study of the immune systems of college students was one of the first to try to document in detail how psychotherapy might lead to better physical health through overcoming people's stoicism and suppression of emotions. However, the idea that repression and suppression of negative feelings may lead to health problems is an old one. It underlies much of Freudian psychotherapy, in which patients work on uncovering traumas hidden in their unconscious. It also underlies theories of biological imbalance, in which the holding back of natural feelings is thought to produce a biological distortion that leads directly to organic dysfunction.

Sue, Jane, and Michelle are three phlegmatic women whose stories surprised me. On the surface, they seemed to be normal, everyday types of people living usual lives, but unfortunate enough to develop serious disease (one had breast cancer, one melanoma, and the third arthritis). Further investigation revealed that Sue had been sexually abused as a child, Jane was living with an alcoholic husband, and Michelle had lost a child in an auto accident. Each of these women reported that she was resigned to a passive life without happiness.

To a casual observer, apathy may not seem so bad. Sue and Michelle had pleasant associations with their neighbors and coworkers. Apathetic, phlegmatic people may appear compliant, unassertive, and even appeasing and cooperative. But they would not be good candidates for close friends.

Phlegmatics do not report being very anxious. They are out of touch with the emotional disturbances in their own bodies. But their hidden feelings can be observed in their closed body positions, their protectively crossed arms or legs, and their tense, submissive movements.

One young college student we assessed in our videotape studies of personality, emotions, and health was a troubling case to contemplate. She revealed a desire to get on and accomplish things in her life, but she felt powerless, alienated, and externally controlled. Although she showed absolutely no signs of outward hostility or aggression either in person or on psychological tests, she harbored high levels of inner anger and hostility. She looked stiff but not sad. Her health already had begun to deteriorate—she suffered from allergies, frequent migraines, and diarrhea. She reminded me very much of some older women who had developed heart disease at an early age.

Some apathetic people share some characteristics with depressed people. Both may have a sense of hopelessness about them. But there are also large differences. Depressed people feel sad or worthless. Apathetic people are not sad. In fact, they often profess to be quite content. Cold, dull, sluggish, cool, and calm are better descriptors. As one writer put it a century ago, "the phlegmatic person is no more easily moved by medicinal than by other agencies."

In the late 1930s, the psychologist Bruno Bettelheim was imprisoned in Dachau, the Nazi concentration camp. (This was before concentration camps officially became death camps.) Bettelheim noticed that certain prisoners soon came to believe that they had no hope of ever leaving the camp alive. They were so emotionally exhausted that they gave the environment complete control over their actions, and they became walking corpses. As Bettelheim put it, "These walking shadows all died very soon."

The psychological transformation affecting most prisoners progressed mostly as follows. First, there was the extreme shock of being uprooted from one's community and placed in an isolated, totally controlled camp environment. Second, there was physical deprivation, involving little sleep, inadequate food, and physical exhaustion. Third, there was psychological harassment—attacks on the prisoners' self-esteem. Witnessing assorted atrocities was not uncommon. Bettelheim kept his own sanity (and his health) by studying the other prisoners.

These manipulations bear an uncanny resemblance to those described by the Russian author Aleksandr Solzhenitsyn in *The Gulag Archipelago*, his book about the prisons and purges of Stalinism. People suddenly were arrested in the middle of the night, dragged off to some prison cell, deprived of food and rest, and physically and mentally taunted and abused. The point of these actions was to make the prisoner lose all sense of feeling, all sense of outrage, compassion, sorrow. These prisoners did not become sad and depressed, they simply turned dull and uncaring. When a prisoner is able to resist such pressures and retain a sense of humanity, we revere him or her as a true modern hero.

Taking a more biological tack, another aspect of the difference between apathy and depression is illustrated by the actions of certain drugs. These drugs, called "catecholamine-depleting drugs" and "cholinergic agonists," interfere with the actions of the body's arousing ("sympathetic") nervous system. It was expected that when given such drugs, people would become depressed. But for many people, this is not the case; instead they become apathetic or sedated. In other words, they are calmed down but do not develop any obvious depressed mood. It is a different emotional state.

In short, when some people experience challenges or disruptions in their lives, they do not react with any overt emotions. Perhaps they have experienced such severe emotional traumas previously that they are no longer able to react. Perhaps they lost control over their lives and resigned themselves to a random existence. Or perhaps as children they never had the close relationships necessary to form emotional attachments. For whatever reason, these people still may be stressed when challenged by happenings in their environment, but they react either without emotion or with well-suppressed emotion. As we shall see, there are serious effects on their health.

WHAT IS DEPRESSION?

Everyone gets sad from time to time; sadness is one of the seven or eight basic emotions that are found in people of all ages, everywhere in the world. Sometimes we say we feel depressed when we feel sad. But depression is more severe than these minor, normal fluctuations in mood.

Truly depressed people have many or most of the following symp-toms: They generally feel sad, down in the dumps; not much makes them happy. They feel tired, weak, indecisive, and worthless but may be very alert to problems. They do not eat or sleep much—or, because a dysregulation is involved, they may eat or sleep too much. But they do not engage in bizarre behaviors or hear voices. In short, they are chronically sad and disturbed but not crazy. The Greeks called such people "melancholic."

Melancholics speak softly, sigh often, and look weak or tired. They may walk with their body slumped, their eyes downcast, and their heads bowed. They have little zest for living. They do things slowly, often with a sad face.

A classic case of depression is described by Emil Kraepelin, the turn-of-the-century German psychiatrist who helped found the mod-ern classification of mental disorders. Kraepelin presents the case of a farmer, a fifty-nine-year-old man who is quite coherent but looks extremely dejected. When questioned, this patient breaks into lamen-tations, claiming that he is apprehensive, wretched, and anxious. He complains of headaches, stomachaches, and insomnia. He thinks about suicide. He groans, trembles, and begs for assistance. Most depressed people are not as bad off as this farmer, but his case nicely captures the essence of this emotionally imbalanced state in its extreme form.

Interestingly, for a psychiatrist to make a diagnosis of depression, so-called organic disorders must be ruled out. The psychiatrist must make sure that the patient does not have hepatitis; the flu; mono-nucleosis; brain or nerve cancer; anemia; blood poisoning; a neuro-logical disorder, such as Parkinson's disease; or a hormonal disorder, such as hypothyroidism or Cushing's syndrome, since all of these conditions and others can produce symptoms of depression. In other words, the traditional medical model of disease forces the physician to separate so-called psychiatric problems from so-called medical prob-lems. So a causal link between depression and illness is not likely to be observed.

The reason for this forced separation is obvious. Sometimes the depression is cured simply by curing the associated disease. For exam-ple, as one defeats the virus and recovers from mononucleosis, one's mood will improve. The problem is that this forced separation between physical and mental states also turns our attention away from the influences of the depression on the medical condition. For example, the depression may be inhibiting recovery from the mononucleosis.

Cushing's syndrome is a medical disorder that often involves a tumor of the pituitary gland, the body's master gland. The main problem that results is an oversupply of cortisol (hydrocortisone), a steroid essential to life. Too much cortisol leads to all sorts of problems, including bodily weakness and the wasting away of muscles. There may be sleep disturbances, eating disorders, a weakening of the immune system, and tremendous fatigue.

The details of the internal regulation of the body are very complex, but one does not have to be an endocrinologist or a neurologist to gain some understanding of the relevant physiological aspects. Most important is the basic idea of homeostasis. The thoughts and feelings of the brain lead to the activation of nerves and hormones throughout the body, and this nerve and hormone activity in turn feeds back to the brain, thus affecting thoughts and feelings. The cortisol found in Cushing's syndrome is released (in most cases) because of a *breakdown* in one piece of this cyclic process, like a broken faucet that cannot be turned off even though the tub is full.

Remarkably, one of the clearest findings in biological psychiatry is that patients with major depression have very high levels of cortisol, sometimes even as high as patients with Cushing's syndrome! This is very significant evidence that depression is closely related to the general mechanisms the body uses to maintain health and internal homeostasis.

Let us go back to Walter Cannon's fight-or-flight response for a minute. Imagine that you are being stalked by a predator and will need to fight or flee. Where would you want to conserve energy in your body? In other words, which internal systems would you want to shut down so that your muscles could work at their best and your body could remain hyperalert? Well, you wouldn't want to worry about eating right, sleeping soundly, engaging in sexual activity, or healing an inflammation. Instead, fearful and worried, you would search for the danger. What would happen if these reactions continued over a long period of time—that is, became chronic? In short, you would be depressed.

In other words, in the case of depression, the best-studied emotional disorder, there is clear evidence that it is closely related to excessive challenge—that is, excessive stress—which manifests itself in a disruption of those internal hormonal systems that generally are used to maintain internal homeostasis. Crucial systems are stretched so far that they go out of whack. Interestingly, as further evidence of this type of systems breakdown, it should be emphasized that some depressed patients do *not* avoid eating, sleeping, and so on, but rather show the exact opposite pole of the disruption—they eat too much, sleep too much, and are not at all vigilant.

Of course, we again face the chicken-or-the-egg issue that is so common in the area of personality and health. Is depression affecting our hormonal balance and general homeostasis, thus resulting in high levels of cortisol? Or are high levels of cortisol leading to depression?

Probably, both processes are occurring. Depression results from too much stress (including stress from challenge and from illness) in susceptible people, and depressed people have an internal imbalance that predisposes them to all sorts of other health problems, including an inability to cope with challenge. This kind of reciprocal relationship is not likely to be detected by a traditional medical approach.

WHAT IS ENTHUSIASM?

The Greek physician Galen left an unresolved problem in his scheme of four humors. Although balance was the essence of the system, three of the humors (choler, melancholy, and phlegm) were seemingly pathological, while the fourth (blood) was healthy. There is an imbalance. A similar issue of asymmetry exists today. What is the opposite of depression, anger, and apathy? Is it simply the absence of these negative states? Is it something positive in its own right? Is it of similar conceptual nature to these others?

These questions are addressed in more detail later. For now it is useful to think of the sanguine (blood) humor as representing cheerfulness and enthusiasm. I like the word *enthusiasm* because it literally means "possessed with the divine spirit." I also like the word *cheer*, because it refers to the "expression of good spirits." As we shall see, this comes close to capturing the essence of the healing personality.

Curiosity and interest are major but often overlooked psychological states. Put in terms of motivation, there is good evidence that people have a basic need to explore their world. A classic and easy-to-recognize case of curiosity involves the responses of a six-month-old child when a shiny new object appears. In adults, an intense level of interest is often reported as "fascination." However, there is also good evidence that this intrinsic motivation can be undermined. People learn to be more or less interested and involved with the world.

Enthusiastic people often are happy and successful in accomplishing tasks or helping other persons, coping well with challenge. They are alert, responsive, and energetic. They walk and talk smoothly and directly, with natural smiles and good eye contact. They tend to touch others more and "reach out" successfully to others. In one study of voice tone, it was shown that the lowest pitch of the voice (called the "fundamental frequency floor") clearly increases under stress in melancholic or phlegmatic people but is relatively unchanged in sanguines. We literally can hear differences in people's responses to challenge.

One young man we studied appeared especially sanguine. Personality tests revealed that Chuck was quite outgoing and not at all hostile, anxious, or depressed. He felt a moderate sense of control over his life and little or no sense of alienation. He smiled naturally and appeared uninhibited and calm when his nonverbal style was analyzed on videotape. Untrained observers reported that Chuck looked especially healthy (and he was in fact in excellent health). Systematic analysis of his body movements showed that he looked friendly and expressive, but not excessively so. He possessed a healthy equilibrium. Interestingly, although likely to remain healthy for the most part, this young man occasionally suffered from allergies—reminding us that we cannot ignore genetic makeup in studying the effects of personality on health.

We all know the experience of happiness, but we do not always think about what it involves. Basically, happiness involves a sense of confidence, security, and good relations with others. Happiness is associated with high levels of love, competence, and optimism. These conclusions are not merely pop philosophizing. They are based on a number of studies showing discrete facial expressions, physiological reactions, and motivational states associated with happiness.

Enthusiastic, sanguine people like Chuck are low on neuroticism. That is, they are calm, relaxed, and secure. But enthusiasm also contains a basic element of personality that is totally separate from neuroticism: "extroversion." Extroverts are sociable, affectionate, spontaneous, fun loving, talkative, and warm. They generally like other people and enjoy the company of others. As we shall see, these various characteristics are important for understanding why some people stay healthy.

Disease-prone Personalities

Let's get right to a key question: Is personality related to dying from cancer? An affirmative answer was suggested in the 1940s by Dr. Franz Alexander, a leading proponent of psychosomatic medicine. He described the cases of two women with breast cancer, both widows, both middle-aged. Two years after mastectomy, Ginny was dying, but Celia was back at her job, with new responsibilities.

Dr. Alexander could not find a biological explanation for the different outcomes, so he sought a psychological one. He found that Ginny was ostentatiously brave and repeatedly asserted that she was going to get well. But she also seemed unable to face her disease or her feelings about losing her breast. Celia, on the other hand, showed neither excessive optimism nor despair. She admitted that losing a breast was hard and tried to find out how she could adjust. She made a remarkable recovery.

Such stories are the hit of cocktail parties, advice columns, and tele-evangelists. Are they true? Can Dr. Alexander's interpretation be supported by hard scientific evidence? In an effort to find out, one recent study at Yale administered psychological questionnaires to fifty-two women with breast cancer. The women's health was then followed for about two years. The results did indeed show that the spread of cancer was greater among women who had a repressed personality, felt hopeless, and seemed unable to express negative emotions.

Only fans of dense technical reports would want to peruse this study. It includes a slew of control variables and design checks—the logical and statistical tools that social scientists use to rule out alternative explanations for the findings. For example, various relevant criteria, such as original disease state and other physiological factors, were taken into account (that is, controlled statistically). Blood counts and related measures ruled out initial physiological differences among the women.

Such features strengthen our ability to draw causal inferences—that is, to conclude that personality played a role in cancer survival. They represent an important improvement over earlier, weaker studies of personality and disease.

The Yale study, for all its statistical sophistication, was only the latest in a long series of studies linking personality to cancer progression. One similar recent study followed 133 premenopausal Canadian women with breast cancer. After initial treatment (usually surgery), the women filled out psychological assessment questionnaires and then were followed for four years. Those women who were more extroverted and who engaged more in social interactions with others were more likely to survive and to remain disease-free.

This is not to suggest that patients can simply wish away their cancer. Cancer is the biological process of cell division gone berserk. Pleasant thoughts may produce miracles for Peter Pan, but they cannot produce miraculous cures. On the other hand, we have seen that there is good reason to believe that psychosocial responses can play an important role in staying healthy.

A interesting example concerns the case of Sue, a young woman who developed malignant melanoma. Melanoma, the most dangerous type of skin cancer, has become increasingly common in recent years, perhaps due to the increase in leisure-time suntanning. Sue fit a typical skin cancer pattern—a blond, light-skinned woman living in a southern climate, with a family history of melanoma. In her twenties, she developed several melanoma growths on her hands and face. All were removed surgically. But Sue's doctors were guarded in their prognosis, worried that the cancer might have spread.

Sue also fit a typical psychosocial profile—she had been a phlegmatic teenager, quietly repressing the turmoil of adolescence. Fortunately, just as the melanoma was discovered, her psychological and social life had begun to change. She had moved out of her parents' home and away from their strict discipline. Her sense of "release" had led her to act quite sociably, and she met a new boyfriend (whom she later married). She also found a program of graduate study that gave her a great sense of personal fulfillment. Ten years after the skin cancer, Sue was still cancer-free. Did the restoration of emotional balance ensure her recovery? For her individual case, we have no way of knowing; but for skin cancer in general, there is evidence that emotional factors can affect the body's defenses.

Other reasonably solid evidence further suggests that depression, repressed anger, or other negative emotions may be relevant to the progression of cancer. Sometimes these feelings are apparent to a casual observer; sometimes they are hidden. In other words, some people who appear strangely easygoing and calm actually may be holding back internal conflicts. A well-known research project in this area was begun in the 1970s. The researchers first studied women hospitalized for a breast biopsy. They then followed up on those diagnosed as having breast cancer. Overall, those women who had internal emotional conflicts (such as repressed anger) and who responded to breast cancer with a stoic and hopeless attitude were more likely to die earlier. At the ten-year follow-up, 55 percent of those who had showed a fighting spirit were still alive, compared to only 22 percent of those who had reacted with a stoic acceptance or a loss of hope.

NKs

Sometimes scientists choose a great name for their scientific discoveries. One of my favorites is "natural killer cells." We are born with these cells, which are part of the immune system that protects us from viruses and other abnormalities. Our natural killer cells find and kill virus-infected cells and cancer cells, just as their name proclaims. (An alternative designation might have been "search-and-destroy" cells.) Ill people with higher levels of natural killer cell activity tend to do better in fighting their illness. Alas, scientists have taken to calling them "NK cells."

These natural killer cells are now the focus of intense research. For example, during the past decade, Dr. Sandra Levy, a tenacious worker, has been laboring at the National Cancer Institute and the University of Pittsburgh to try to understand the precise role of psychobiology in breast cancer. In one study of women with advanced cancer, she found that along with several biological factors, a psychological dimension of good feelings and vigor termed "joy" was a good predictor of longer survival. Sure enough, a second study found that patients who lacked close ties with other people and who were listless and apathetic tended to have lower levels of NK cell activity. Such studies are important because they are starting to reveal the biological mechanisms that account for the effects of personality on health.

An interesting twist was provided by a study of lung cancer in 224 men and women. Lung cancer is a relatively easy cancer for personality researchers to study, since most victims are dead within a year or two. This particular study followed patients who had been diagnosed within only the past few months. As expected (on the basis of biological understanding of lung cancer), most of the patients had died by the end of one year. As expected (on the basis of psychological understanding of disease susceptibility), those patients with a reserved (as opposed to outgoing) personality were more likely to have died. The twist was that also more likely to die were patients whose personality was either much more sober *or* much more enthusiastic than average. This study thus implies that one can have too much of a good thing— be too optimistic and enthusiastic—and reminds us again of the importance of internal balance.

WHAT ABOUT CANCER DEVELOPMENT?

The evidence just reviewed concerned the prognosis of people who already had cancer. What about the effects of personality on health *before* people get cancer? Does personality play a role in causing cancer?

To address these questions, an important large-scale study examined the health of about two thousand men whose personality had been measured back in 1958. The men were all employees of the Western Electric company in Chicago. At that time (late 1950s), some of the men scored high on a measure of depression and poor social relations. That is, they responded to questionnaire items that indicated that they were unhappy, sensitive to criticism, of low self-worth, prone to disturbed sleep, unsociable, and so on.

During the next twenty years, these depressed men were more likely than the other men to die of cancer. Importantly, this increased risk remained even after the researchers took into account the men's age, cigarette smoking, occupation, and family history of cancer. Of course, many of the depressed men did not develop cancer, but depression was a definite risk factor. In addition, the depressed men also were somewhat more likely than the nondepressed men to die of noncancer causes. Depression was a general risk factor for early death.

An interesting footnote to this Western Electric study concerns changes over time. The longer the time since the measurement of depression, the weaker the association to illness and death. One interpretation of this trend is that emotional problems at one point in time will not necessarily have an effect far into the future. Some of the men in the sample might have overcome their depression during those twenty years, thus reducing the threat to their health. These matters are considered further in the discussion of changing disease proneness in chapter 8.

Is the Western Electric study the only evidence of this sort? Not at all. A different study was based at the Johns Hopkins University School of Medicine. Called the "Precursors Study," this research began studying male medical students in 1948. Upon entering medical school, students were asked about their personality and family relations. Researchers found that during the following thirty years, those physicians who seemed to have social and emotional problems were more likely to develop cancer.

Another interesting, albeit controversial, research program was begun in Yugoslavia by a psychologist named Ronald Grossarth-Maticek. This research has reported close relationships between certain aspects of personality and subsequent death from cancer or heart disease, including the finding that hopelessness and repression of emotions leads to an increased likelihood of cancer. However, the findings of this study were so clear and so strong that many scientists in this field are skeptical. In the coming years, experienced scientists will attempt to repeat this research. In this book, I present only those studies that I have evaluated and concluded to be carefully designed, well conducted, and convincing. I have not come to any conclusion about the research of Grossarth-Maticek, although his findings are consistent with many of my own assertions.

Recently I have heard people remark, "If you don't get heart disease, then you'll get cancer." This statement derives from a finding that cholesterol levels in the blood may be inversely (negatively) related to the incidence of cancer; so the lower the cholesterol, the greater the likelihood of cancer. However, there are a number of reasons that may account for such an association that do not imply that a low level of cholesterol in the blood *causes* cancer. All in all, the evidence regarding cholesterol and cancer is much too tentative to make claims regarding this intriguing finding. It is, however, consistent with the idea that metabolic irregularities at either extreme are a link between personality and disease.

Not every study of cancer finds a relationship to personality. Some find no relationship at all, especially those that study personality and the development of cancer (as opposed to its progression). It is important not to overlook these inconsistent findings. It would be an oversimplification to say that personality problems cause cancer. But there is enough evidence that personality plays a role in cancer for researchers to begin to think with some confidence about a cancer-prone personality. However, there is no clear evidence proving that the various *emotional reactions* that are relevant to cancer are radically different from those that predispose a person to other diseases as well.

The remainder of this chapter provides a complete and up-to-date analysis of the role of personality factors in disease. But first let us briefly sum up what is known regarding personality and cancer:

It seems that most forms of cancer are more likely to develop as a result of problems with one's genes or one's environment than as a result of emotional problems. If you smoke, breathe polluted air, are exposed to radiation, eat contaminated food or water, suntan regularly, or otherwise damage your body's cells, or if you chose the wrong parents, you greatly increase your risk of cancer. To the extent that personality problems make it more likely that one will engage in smoking or unhealthy behaviors, then emotional problems are a cause, though an indirect cause, of cancer. There also may very well be some direct risk of cancer for emotionally troubled persons, but this risk is not huge; it has appeared only in certain studies.

On the other hand, there is good evidence—including evidence from animal studies—that emotions do affect survival once cancer begins to develop. People who are poorly adjusted, have given up hope, and have disturbed interpersonal relations are less likely to succeed in their battle against cancer. And, as we shall see, negative emotions play an important role in many other diseases as well.

Some news accounts pretend that the notion that negative emotions can play a role in the progression of cancer is controversial and not real science. Traditional medicine is wary of psychosocial influences, and some reports may act as if these matters are at the fringes of scientific medicine. In fact, the evidence of the role of personality and stress in the progression of disease is fairly substantial for cancer and, as we shall see, overwhelming for cardiovascular disease.

TYPE A, TYPE B, AND ALPHABET SOUP: A NEW PERSPECTIVE ON HEART DISEASE

In the 1950s, two cardiologists, Meyer Friedman and Ray Rosenman, noticed some interesting relationships between personality and heart disease. When an upholsterer arrived to repair the chairs in their office waiting room, he asked them what kinds of physicians they were. The upholsterer wondered why only the front edges of the chairs were worn out. It seemed that their heart patients were especially likely to sit on the edge of their seats! Although not scientific proof, this incident suggested a possible link between persistently agitated behavior and heart disease.

The cardiologists began a systematic study of the disturbed psychological patterns they saw in their patients. They named the phenomenon the "Type A behavior pattern." The term *Type A* sounded new, unique, and scientific, but it was probably a poor choice. The problem is that Type A is such a neutral term that its definition can be subtly changed through sleight of hand. Ask ten doctors to define Type A and you will get ten different definitions. Fortunately, recent research by myself and others has helped explain what Type A behavior is all about.

How did its originators view the Type A personality? Type A

people have been perceived, for the most part, as those involved in a constant struggle to do more and more things in less and less time, and who are sometimes quite aggressive in their efforts to achieve them. Type A people were seen as always under the pressure of time, suffering a "hurry sickness" of constantly having a deadline to meet.

In many cases Type A behavior can be easily and reliably diagnosed. A couple of years ago, in the course of interviewing a Type A man, we asked him whether he plays tennis for the fun of it or in order to win. He shouted back, "*I play to kill!*" Such extreme Type A individuals live a life characterized by intense competitiveness; they are always striving for dominance.

The idea that emotional factors can play a role in the health of the heart is of course an old one. Literature is full of references to links among the heart, personality, and emotions. For example, here are two biblical sayings: "A happy heart cheers the countenance but a sad heart is a depressed spirit" (Prov. 15:13). "Gladness of the heart is the life of a man, and the joy of a man prolongs his days" (Apoc. 30:22). In fact, today the term "broken heart" refers not to a ruptured muscle or a malfunctioning valve, but to an emotional state that pervades the body and spirit.

In the 1930s, the Menninger brothers and other psychiatrists began to claim that cardiovascular disease in general and heart disease in particular were associated with excessive competitiveness and aggressiveness. For example, Dr. Franz Alexander, the mid-century leader in psychosomatic medicine who presented the breast cancer example of Ginny and Celia, describes the case of a man with severe and fluctuating high blood pressure. This man appeared polite, retiring, and self-conscious, but at the same time he was very ambitious to excel. As a boy, he had been overaggressive and domineering, but pressures from his father and his social environment had turned him overtly inhibited and unexpressive. Dr. Alexander related these aggressive, rebellious tendencies directly to the man's blood pressure.

So, the invention of the Type A pattern by cardiologists in the 1950s was nothing new, but it did do something special: it led to rigorous scientific studies to test this formulation. The Type A personality has now been studied for more than thirty years. But many accounts of Type A in the popular press (and in doctors' offices) are at least ten years behind the evidence.

Type A Evidence

The best evidence linking Type A behavior to heart disease comes from a study called the Western Collaborative Group study. Starting in 1960, about three thousand working men were assessed on a variety of physical and mental health measures. Only men who were initially free of heart disease were included in the study. Through a personal interview, the men were diagnosed as either Type A or Type B. (The interview assessment is important because it allows measurement of emotional style.) After about eight years, the Type A men were found to be more than twice as likely as the Type B men to have developed heart disease. This link held when other traditional risk factors were taken into account.

This connection was confirmed by two other long-term prospective studies. The famous Framingham (Massachusetts) study is the long-term research program from which we have gotten most of our best information about the role of diet, cholesterol, and other risk factors in heart disease; it also found an effect of being Type A. Similar findings come from a European study called the French-Belgian Collaborative Heart Study, which followed working men in Brussels, Marseilles, and Paris. The link between Type A and heart disease also has been found in dozens of studies in which heart disease patients have been examined in terms of their personality characteristics.

However, as in the case of most links between personality and illness, the relationship is not always confirmed. News reports may trumpet these occasional failures. This state of affairs has left some people skeptical and has encouraged many physicians to disparage the whole topic, especially since some were predisposed against thinking about psychosocial matters in the first place.

Interestingly, a sort of polarization has developed in the practice of cardiology. The original proponents of the Type A concept (who have long since split into their own ideological camps) sometimes seem to be defending Type A to the bitter end while under assault from their more biomedically minded colleagues, who would just as soon stick with their angiograms and forget about psychology altogether.

This scientific tension is apparent in the insightful writings of Norman Cousins. Cousins, former editor of the *Saturday Review*, retreated to California to continue writing and to work as an adjunct professor of medicine at the University of California, Los Angeles, where he tried to humanize medical care. Cousins writes of the difficulties faced even by a famous and influential person like himself in trying to relieve the oppressive technical climate of the medical system. During his own heart attack, Cousins worked to convince his doctors that they should be paying more attention to the environmental and emotional influences on his health—including the atmosphere in the cardiac care unit and the heart testing centers. Shortly after being wheeled into the hospital, he asked the cardiologist if it was okay for him to do some writing.

Later Cousins was able to listen to Bach and Beethoven recordings during a treadmill test. He was sure his heart would pump better in the right emotional climate. (But I wouldn't suggest trying this yourself, unless you are willing to have some very strange psychiatric notations written in your medical chart!)

The case reports described by Cousins and others do not constitute scientific evidence. However insightful, they are just individual testimonials. Fortunately, scientific evidence for understanding this matter does exist.

The state of affairs I have just described is about as far as most lay people have followed the matter. Most people have heard about the Type A personality but are not sure about its implications. Does Type A behavior really cause coronary heart disease? Do other aspects of personality cause heart disease? I have been studying these issues for a number of years, using two approaches. First, I have applied newly developed statistical methods to reanalyze dozens of previous studies involving thousands of people. Second, I have studied Type A people in my own laboratory. What have I found?

Basically, there is ample evidence that certain aspects of personality (related to being Type A) do indeed predispose certain people to heart disease. But the critical characteristics are not the ones people usually associate with heart disease.

Pathological Competition
and Toxic Hostility

As I moved around over the years, I have had checking accounts at banks in New York, Boston, and several cities in southern California. On many occasions in southern California, I have walked into a bank to cash a check and found myself to be the sole customer, or perhaps one of only two or three customers. Still, it often has taken fifteen minutes before I was finished and could leave the bank. In New York or Boston, I have seen banks handle fifty or more customers in less than fifteen minutes.

Sure enough, heart disease rates are generally lower in the southern and western United States than in the fast-paced large cities of the northeast. But it would be a mistake to conclude (as many people do) that the fast pace causes disease. In fact, people like myself, who have experience with efficient banks and who become frustrated in slow-paced banks, are probably better off dealing with Boston banks.

Originally Type A was defined very broadly, describing an active, hard-working, hurrying, hostile, tense, and impatient person. However, the inconsistent nature of research findings on Type A has led to refining the concept. In other words, since only some measures of Type A personality in some populations are found to be related to heart disease, it makes sense that certain aspects may be more relevant than others.

The first clue about where to look was provided in 1977 by a study that reexamined data from the Western Collaborative Group research. This study found that the single element that contributed the most to the relationship between Type A and heart disease was "potential for hostility." Since hostility was long suspected as a factor in coronary disease proneness, attention rapidly turned toward this component.

At that point, several studies began to confirm that a hostility scale (called the Cook-Medley scale) predicted coronary heart disease. It also predicted coronary atherosclerosis, the process of plaque-based hardening of the arteries that supply the heart muscle with blood.

A few years ago, we interviewed a seemingly friendly and courteous sixty-two-year-old man, Joe, who was recovering from a massive heart attack. Despite the fact that the heart attack had forced a number of improvements in this man's life-style, he turned out to be one of the most hostile Type A men we had ever encountered. He practically oozed coronary proneness.

Joe was in the retail business, and he did whatever was necessary to make a buck. Joe had often worked long hours, always for the money. He viewed life as a competitive struggle for dominance. For example, if forced to wait for a table in a restaurant, he would go over to the hostess with a fifty-dollar bill and demand immediate seating. He would tap the hostess on the shoulder, slip the fifty dollars into her hand, look her straight in the eye, smile broadly, and announce, "My name is Joe and I have an important business meeting that requires immediate seating."

Joe continuously interrupted our interviewer, explaining and justifying his answers. Occasionally his hands formed into fists. In an effort to control his aggressiveness, he often sighed deeply, an unsuccessful attempt to appear calm.

This man's social relations were poor. When asked whether he had played with his children when they were young, Joe furrowed his brow and replied, "No, but I should have." He said his wife found him hard to deal with: "I have a temper." When asked whether he was more aggressive than his peers, he answered insightfully, "No, I don't think so, but then again, most of them are dead."

Joe's problem was not that he was ambitious, or that he worked long hours, or even that he had a bad temper. Rather, it was his overwhelmingly choleric patterns that soured his relationships, and attacked his equilibrium, and contributed to his ill health.

The recent scientific evidence is sufficient to conclude that hostility, born of excessive competition, rather than "hurry-sickness," is a prime component of Type A personality and a reliable independent predictor of heart disease. That is, it is unhealthy to be a person who generally responds to frustrating circumstances with anger, irritation, and disgust. Interestingly, hostility also seems to be a good predictor of death from all causes. But, contrary to what some people think, hostility is *not* the only relevant factor.

Type B and Phony Type B

My wife had an uncle named Sam who was very active and alert in his mid-eighties. He would go for walks even in winter on icy streets in not-so-tame big city neighborhoods. His philosophy was "I try my best, and I trust in God." He never participated in a study of heart disease, but if he had, he would have been diagnosed as Type B.

In addition to the high heart disease rates in most northeastern cities, the states in the eastern third of the United States have higher rates of heart disease than do the western states. The Rocky Mountain states—Idaho, Montana, Utah, Wyoming, and New Mexico—have especially low rates. No one knows for sure why this is the case, but a good guess is that the difference is at least partly due to something about the more easygoing life-style of those in the West.

Heart disease was rare as the twentieth century began, but then it emerged rapidly in the industrialized West. Part of the reason for increased rates of heart disease is that people today are no longer dying young from infectious diseases like smallpox. But this explanation alone cannot account for the tremendous rise in cardiovascular disease rates and for the fact that various segments of our populations are still not at high risk.

Some of the difference in disease rates can be explained by variations in diet, in smoking habits, and in genetic background. But that leaves a great deal to be explained. The explanation is differences in personality: people with a disease-resistant personality are able to avoid heart disease.

The traditional medical approach to health leads us to define things backward—that is, in a negative way. This is easiest to see in medical testing. If you have a blood test, or a urine test, or an X ray, the good result is that the test is "negative." In other words, nothing was found to be abnormal. This is an endless source of confusion to patients, who are used to thinking of the default state as being positive, not negative—and so they are distressed by a negative result. In any other situation, a negative test result is bad news. But in medicine, good is defined as the absence of bad.

This same backward approach has been applied to defining Type B, or the non-coronary-prone personality. Type B has simply been viewed as the absence of Type A behaviors. So people are told what they should not do, but not what they *should* do. Can Type B be defined in its own right?

My own research in this area suggests that a true Type B person is comfortable and relaxed, open and friendly. Although not hostile, these healthy people are not at all submissive. They are even healthy-looking. They are calm and cheerful rather than anxious and depressed.

Sy was a sixty-year-old man with no signs of heart disease or any other major health problems. Aside from a touch of hay fever, he was the picture of good health. Married for thirty-five years, Sy had lived in the same geographic area for forty years, and he had many friends and acquaintances.

Contrary to what some people might imagine, Sy was in no way an inert bump on a log. A retired police lieutenant, Sy had worked in an inherently stressful position. He had always felt under pressure when working, but, he told us, "I didn't get too emotionally involved; I wasn't bothered by it. That was what I did, so I worked it out as best I could." Not only that, but Sy had worked two jobs for a while, always remaining healthy.

In retirement, Sy built furniture. He reported, "My leisure time is spent working on things I like to do. Gives me a feeling of accomplishing something—I do it for self-satisfaction and for other people." His life was certainly not boring and slow-paced. He always worked quickly but planned ahead. He was even somewhat impatient—for example, he told us he generally would not wait at a restaurant for a table. But if he did wait, he would talk with his associates and the wait would not bother him.

When Sy had an appointment, he was always on time; if others were late, he would come right out and ask, "Why the hell weren't you here?" Sy told us that he played games for the fun of it. "But," he smiled, "of course, winning makes it a little better."

Sy spoke slowly and with a slight drawl (he was originally from Kentucky), in a deep, expressive, Ronald Reagan–type tone. Sometimes during the interview, there were long periods before he responded to questions; he never interrupted. He said he had strong feelings at times, and he generally revealed them: "When I'm angry, you know it. I would yell a bit in my younger days." But he usually maintained a sense of equilibrium and perspective. For example, when rushed, he would remind himself, "What the heck, the world's not going to end if I don't finish this."

In short, Sy led a challenging life, but one that he liked and could handle. He had a realistic approach to difficulty, at one point saying "there is no Shangri-la." His sense of humor was readily apparent, even in a brief encounter.

Unfortunately, there are many people who look like Sy superficially but are actually at high risk for health problems. My research has uncovered what I call *phony Type Bs*. These people may, at first glance, appear to be Type B. That is, they do not rush around or compete aggressively. But their extreme competitive drive is hidden just below the surface. They may remain stuck in a middle-level job. They are tense, powerless, and alienated, although you may not see this unless you looked carefully. Many are phlegmatic. Just like the hostile, choleric Type As, they are prone to disease.

One such phlegmatic man we interviewed spoke very calmly and deliberately about his job. There were few signs of problems until he was asked whether he desired to move up in the company. He answered, "Oh, sure, I feel I can achieve much more." Further exploration revealed that he was quite tense and alienated because he felt that his abilities were not being recognized. He was not a Type A or choleric, but he was at high risk for ill health.

Another phony Type B man we studied was a real mess in terms of health. Sixty-five years old and retired, Roger previously had worked in construction. He had chest pain, breathing problems, and fainting spells and had recently had pneumonia and a minor stroke. Like Sy, Roger had lived in the same town for many years. But he was not satisfied there; he said that he would like to live in Hawaii, although he had never been there.

Roger looked and sounded tense, although he genuinely tried to be friendly. His parents had separated when he was young (an unusual occurrence in those days), and that seemed to have been a significant problem for him in his relations with others. Concerning stress, Roger said that pressure did not bother him, but then he agreed that "nobody likes to be under pressure." When angry, he said he would not explode; instead he held it in. He did woodworking as a hobby, which gave him a sense of control and relaxed him. He tended to be a perfectionist in his work.

On psychological testing, Roger was found to be anxious and somewhat depressed. But this was not readily apparent in an interview. He did seem somewhat distracted. When working (before retirement), however, he said he had been very bothered by the unrealistic expectations of his supervisors.

Roger's inner conflicts often manifested themselves in a sense of uncertainty. He was full of ambivalence. Would he wait for a table at a restaurant? "Well, again, it depends." Would he be impatient while waiting? "I'd try not to be."

Roger always kept his appointments. If others were late, he said, "Oh, I might resent it."

This phony Type B never tried to do two things at once. He was slow and calm in many ways, and a pleasant sort of guy. But Roger had an inner dissatisfaction that seemed to exacerbate his health problems.

We also studied a friend of Roger's, a retired U.S. Air Force officer. This man also seemed calm on the surface but was holding in a tremendous amount of anger. He died of a heart attack ten months after the interview.

In the next chapter, we shall consider what might be called the "heart-healthy personality." But for now, let's get away from this Type A, Type B labeling and just call emotional patterns what they are—hostility, depression, relaxation, enthusiasm, or whatever.

Don't Slow Down

Thousands of people are being given bad advice about avoiding heart attacks. They are being told to slow down, to take it easy, to take vacations, and even to retire from their jobs. In fact, there is not a shred of evidence that regular hard work increases the likelihood of heart disease in a healthy person. (A different situation, of course, is a patient with an impaired heart whose doctor has advised strict limits on activity.)

When the comedian George Burns was eighty years old, he said he would never retire. "I think the only reason you should retire is if you can find something you enjoy doing more than what you're doing now. . . . I don't see what age has to do with retirement."

Burns was exactly right. Sociologists have shown that retirement is healthy for some people, unhealthy for others. If retirement allows a person to escape from a frustrating or overwhelming job, then retirement will likely be healthy. If retirement means giving up an interesting daily routine, losing economic status, or moving away from friends, then retirement may be unhealthy. *In other words, it is a terrible (though common) oversimplification to think that health will improve when people retire and "take it easy."* Renowned cellist Pablo Casals put it this way: "To stop, to retire even for a short time, is to begin to die."

As part of my own extensive examination of this topic, I reanalyzed past findings on what has been called "job involvement." This is more psychological jargon to describe the fact that some people seem very committed to and involved in their work. It often has been stated that such hard work is unhealthy. However, when my student Stephanie Booth-Kewley and I looked at all of the evidence, we found no links between job involvement and various measures of heart disease. Hard workers were just as healthy as everyone else.

Many people are mistakenly called coronary prone because they are so dedicated and hardworking. In reality, these busy beavers are likely to be exceptionally healthy if they also are friendly, energetic, and emotionally expressive and feel in control of their lives. This finding is a tremendous relief to my many hardworking colleagues in universities around the country who wonder in the back of their minds whether they should be spending less time in the lab and more time on the beach.

This misunderstanding of the true nature of coronary proneness is also another example of how a misreading of the nature of health can have costly economic implications. We should not be harassing the hardworking, self-fulfilled, and productive members of our society, telling them to slow down. Similarly, we should not be forcing satisfied workers into mandatory retirement (at least not for reasons of their own health). Not only are we in danger of losing these valuable workers from production, but we may be causing them enough frustration to increase their likelihood of illness!

On the other hand, it is counterproductive to pressure those people who are unwilling or unable to succeed at their present line of work. It generally would be more productive and healthier to find them a more suitable work environment. Although this utopian view cannot always be fulfilled, it can be addressed more often than is currently the case.

High Stress, No Exit

Jean-Paul Sartre knew what existential hell was—being trapped with people you despise and having no exit. In our modern society, this entrapment is most likely to be in a job with a hated boss.

With an early interest in physics, I grew up hearing that nature abhors a vacuum. Yet the study of risk factors for disease often assumes that each factor occurs in a vacuum. In fact, of course, each influence on health is affected by the overall context of a person's life. In the case of personality and emotional reactions, they occur in the context of challenging situations.

Many people develop heart disease not because their job is too stressful but because it is too stressful *for them.* A job with high expectations may be unhealthy for an individual with few personal resources, but a job with few demands may likewise be unhealthy for an ambitious and competitive person. It is the match or mismatch that is most important. Furthermore, for most people and most jobs, the demands come not from the job itself but from other people at the job site.

Ask a secretary to choose between a nasty boss with a light workload and a nice boss who imposes a heavy workload; which situation do you think he or she will prefer? Ask a physician what is most stressful about the profession and the answer most likely will concern neither the long hours nor the technical details but the psychological reactions of patients and their families. Ask a middle-level manager about his or her greatest source of frustration and it probably will be the immediate boss, not the amount of desk work. As large American corporations begin to recognize this fact, they start to follow the lead of the Japanese, who strive to improve interpersonal relations and keep their workers feeling contented.

We can go even further. Several studies have indicated a link between belonging to a low social class and having a high risk of heart disease. Other studies have found a higher risk of disease of all sorts among the poor. We could try to isolate the particular factors that cause this poor health—bad nutrition, more cigarette smoking, less access to health care, more substance abuse, more emotional traumas, more exposure to toxic chemicals, less knowledge about prevention, close quarters (contagion), poor prenatal care, daily stresses, substandard shelter, and so on. But I do not think that we could ever pin down the "real" reason. Rather, poor people face a whole series of inter-related challenges in their environment. When economic factors deprive people of the emotional resources needed to deal with the myriad of challenges that everyone faces, the likelihood of illness markedly increases. Their situation is one of high stress, no exit. The problem with the health of poor people is that they are poor.

In sum, there is strong evidence that people who lead hostile, competitive, and driven lives are more likely to suffer heart disease than are more easygoing people. But it is not hard work, activity, or a challenging job that is the problem. Rather, it is the emotional struggle that is the problem.

UNHEALTHY MOTIVATIONAL STATES

When an airplane crashes, killing all of its passengers, the relatives of the victims are of course devastated. Their patterns of emotional reactions are interesting to examine. First, there is generally shock and denial. Then there is terrible sadness and grief. Often this is followed by intense anger—with the airline, with God, and even with the dead victims for having the audacity to die suddenly. Later there is often depression, followed by withdrawal and apathy. Finally, many months or even years later, a more cheerful mood usually returns, although some element of sadness often remains.

What is interesting about these emotional reaction patterns is that they are not distinct; rather, they flow one from the other, and all from the same source. In other words, although anger and apathy and depression seem—and indeed are—different in many ways, they also are linked. When we experience an imbalance or disharmony with our worlds, various significant emotional disorders can result.

I think this insight is too often overlooked in thinking about personality and health. It is a mistake to focus on only one emotional reaction, such as repressed anger. Nevertheless, it is true that different underlying motivations come into play to cause these various reactions. To try to understand in greater detail the causes of emotional disturbance, it is useful to examine briefly the relevant aspects of motivation or striving that people have.

Competitiveness and Irritation

In a utopia man and woman would not have to struggle or toil. Presumably they would not experience any feelings of frustration or irritation either. However, most of us do face challenges that we must strive to conquer. And some of us try harder than others.

Everyone likes to achieve a sense of mastery or competence. Such feelings of control generally are healthy. But people prone to cardiovascular problems (and other diseases) are driven to *excessive* achievement and to total mastery of their worlds. This argument was developed more than a decade ago by Dr. David Glass, one of the first researchers to seriously study the psychological elements of coronary proneness.

In various studies, Dr. Glass showed that Type A people work hard to succeed, refuse to feel tired, and are especially likely to react with hostility when frustrated. In other words, their excessive hostility and competitiveness can be traced to a desire to maintain control. This desire for control is not necessarily bad—in fact, it is a key aspect of good health for most people. (This is examined further in the next chapter.) It is only when the desire is excessive and all-consuming that problems arise.

Other people just never seem to succeed in gaining much control, no matter how hard they try. They strive and strive but lose each time. When I was growing up, my father often pointed out these *schlemazels*. (The *schlemazel* is the person upon whom the waiter always spills the soup.) What happens when competitively driven individuals repeatedly see that they cannot attain their goals? What do they do when they recognize that the situation is beyond their control? These individuals are especially likely to lapse into hopelessness and depression.

Hopelessness

During the Korean War, thousands of American soldiers were captured by the North Koreans. Numerous prisoners, under severe stress in a hostile environment, became apathetic and listless and then died. The other prisoners called it "give up–itis."

If you are a former soldier telling your friends about "give up–itis," most of them will nod and understand what you mean. But if you want to achieve scientific renown and inspire others, you have to develop the idea, cast it into a conceptual framework, and give it a fancy title. Professor Martin Seligman did this in his influential "Theory of Learned Helplessness."

The basic idea is a simple one. Imagine you are in a situation where you cannot control the outcome, no matter what you do—for example, a child who is totally ignored by her parents, an adult in an unbending job, or a person in a scientific laboratory facing uncontrollable noise. The typical outcome of such a situation is that the individual learns to be helpless. That is, the individual will make no effort to control his or her surroundings, even when subsequently placed in a controllable environment. Numerous animal studies have demonstrated that helpless, stressed animals have faster-growing cancer tumors.

What are the psychological consequences of this helplessness? First, the individual simply becomes less active and less motivated. Second, the individual has trouble developing new ways of dealing with the world; learning becomes more difficult. Third, and most important for our purposes, the individual is likely to become depressed. In other words, deeply sad feelings and other aspects of depression begin to take over the person's life. The helplessness turns into hopelessness. For example, in the case of the relatives of a plane crash victim, once all of the anger and the demands and the "why didn't you . . ." questions lead to naught, the relatives simply may give up and collapse into a state of depression.

It is not the loss itself that leads to depression but how we think about the loss. For example, when Candy Lightner's teenage daughter Cari was killed by a drunk driver (a repeat offender), she felt devastated and frustrated. But instead of lapsing into a long-term depression as so many bereaved parents do, she founded Mothers Against Drunk Driving (MADD). This organization not only has been remarkably successful in changing laws and public awareness about drunk driving, but it has proved to be a major asset in protecting the emotional health of many other mothers who have faced the same terrible loss. If you have ever encountered a MADD mother in a shopping mall, you know that she is anything but helpless.

This line of thinking can be taken a step further. We have seen that people who believe they have some control over their lives are less prone to destructive emotional states. However, everyone faces some events (such as their own mortality or that of their parents) that they know they cannot control. Some people are psychologically able to assume that they will be capable of managing their feelings. Others, however, worry that they will not be able to cope when the sad time arrives. That is, what they fear is fear itself. This worry about future worries may lead in turn to distress and harmful nervous system arousal. Some disease-prone people are depressed about becoming depressed.

Suspiciousness, Pessimism, and Cynicism

In the early 1940s, a number of healthy young Harvard undergraduates entered a scientific study. They underwent a physical examination and completed a battery of personality tests. Many of these men were then followed for the next forty years.

In light of recent developments in the area of psychology and health, researchers dug the old questionnaires out of a closet and analyzed responses given by the men in 1946. The responses were categorized as indicating either a negative and pessimistic explanatory style or an optimistic outlook. For example, one pessimistic man wrote, "I have symptoms of fear and nervousness . . . similar to those my mother has had."

What were the relationships to subsequent health? Starting at about age forty-five, a clear difference emerged in the health and longevity of these men: the pessimistic men were less likely to be alive and healthy.

In this kind of study, various links between personality and health (examined in chapter 2) probably are operating. Pessimists are less likely to take care of themselves. They are more likely to place themselves in risky situations. They probably experience more stress, since they view life's challenges with a jaundiced eye. And so on. Unfortunately, we do not know much about the men's habits, so it is impossible to know which influences most affected their health.

A different but kindred study conducted at Duke University and published in 1987 addressed this issue by studying a sample of white middle-class adults. This study used the scores of five hundred older men and women on a personality test called the 16 PF. Part of this test measures suspiciousness, cynicism, and mistrust. It was found that those people who had high scores on suspiciousness were more likely to die during a fifteen-year period. This link between personality and death still existed after the investigators took into account age, smoking history, alcohol history, and cholesterol levels in the blood. So it was not the case that these people increased their disease risk solely by engaging in an number of unhealthy habits. Rather, their suspicious approach to the world seemed unhealthy. In addition, this study found that the presence of suspiciousness increased the likelihood of both cancer and heart disease.

Seeing the importance of the impact of suspicion and cynicism on health, I went back to the older scientific literature, looking for similar evidence. Sure enough, a well-conducted prospective study of middle-aged men published in 1964 had used the same 16 PF test, including the suspiciousness subscale. Which aspect of personality was related to subsequent health? The suspiciousness scale clearly predicted the likelihood of a heart attack. It also predicted who would develop angina (chest pain). To me, such striking convergence of evidence is very convincing.

I am guilty of having oversimplified something earlier in this chapter: The Cook-Medley scale that predicts heart disease does not simply measure hostility. It also assesses aspects of cynicism, mistrust, and alienation. Thus, a suspicious and cynical approach to one's world as well as excessive competition may contribute to the health-damaging feelings of chronic hostility. As the ancient Greeks understood, the choleric humor is related not only to anger but also to bitterness.

About a decade ago, a well-known personality psychologist named Julian Rotter wrote an article about trust that I think has, unfortunately, been overlooked by most psychologists. In it, Dr. Rotter asserts (and presents evidence) that people who trust others are less likely to be unhappy, conflicted, or maladjusted. They are more dependable and have more friends. They are not necessarily more gullible, they are just less cynical. In brief, they are healthier. This is not a moral judgment; it is merely a summary of the empirical evidence. Trust is a motivation directly relevant to the healing personality.

Repression

Tecumseh, Michigan, is a community of about ten thousand middle-class whites. Starting in the late 1950s, the health of this whole community has been studied intermittently by scientists. In 1971, an interesting psychosocial measure was taken on a sample of these residents. The people were asked: "Imagine that your husband (or wife or sweetheart) yelled in anger or blew up at you for something that wasn't your fault." Would you get angry or annoyed and show it? Or would you get angry or annoyed and keep it in, or not get angry at all?

The people were then followed for about a decade, during which time about 8 percent of them died. As expected on the basis of extensive past research, those people (especially men) with high blood pressure, a low educational level, and poorer initial health were more likely to die. However, even after controlling for these effects, repressed anger had a dramatic impact on health. Persons who had said they would hold their anger in were almost two and a half times more likely to die than those who would express their anger to their mate.

What is especially interesting about this study is that it looks not at anger as a cause of heart disease or repression and depression as a cause of cancer, but at repressed anger as a cause of all mortality. Other studies have found the same relationship, although usually they have not interpreted it in this way. These studies complement the research on the risks of hostility. In other words, there is reasonable evidence that it is not just feelings of hostility, repression of anger, or a hopeless depression that leads to a specific problem. Rather, it seems as if patterns of emotional disturbance are unhealthy, period. The ancient Greeks would not have been surprised by these findings.

In the last chapter, we saw that repression of feelings was related to apathy. It turns out that there has been quite a bit of psychological theorizing during the past decade or two about just this topic. Some of this work is on "alexithymia," which literally means "without words for feelings." It has been noticed repeatedly by clinicians that their patients with this condition are especially likely to suffer from diseases thought to have a strong psychosomatic component.

Another way to approach this issue is simply to look at people's emotional expressions. Some people readily show their feelings—these are the open and fascinating people whom most of us like to be around. President Reagan was a good example. He always had just the right tear in his eye or nod of his head. He created trust and empathy in others. On the other hand, many people hold back their feelings and seem inscrutable.

Those of us who study nonverbal emotional expressions have developed reliable means of measuring expressiveness. The basic technique is to videotape people and then apply various standardized judgment techniques to the videotaped expressions. We analyze facial expressions, tone of voice, posture, and body movement.

When one looks at a phlegmatic person on the videotape, there is just no information about what he or she is feeling. The findings regarding health are consistent. The constant holding back of feelings sets in motion a pattern of harmful physiological reactions. People who hold back expression of their feelings are more prone to disease.

In sum, the evidence we have just reviewed comes from several very different psychological approaches. Each study, considered alone, is not so impressive. But when the evidence is laid out together, some very striking patterns appear. It is exciting to see the consistencies; it is this orderliness that convinced me to write this book.

Thus far, we have examined the associations between certain emotional aspects of personality and the two greatest killers—cancer and heart disease. We have traced these harmful emotional reactions to several underlying motivations—hostile competitiveness, helplessness and hopelessness, suspiciousness and pessimism, and repression of feelings. Their links to disease are consistent. But what about other common health problems, such as asthma, migraines, ulcers, and arthritis, as a function of negative emotional states? What about the big picture?

THE BIG PICTURE

As I first began to evaluate scientific studies probing a link between certain aspects of personality and disease, I became more and more confused. One study examined anger and heart disease, the next looked at depression and cancer, a third looked at anxiety and ulcers, and so on. Furthermore, although many of the studies found a link, some did not.

Finally I exclaimed to the graduate students I was supervising, "*What does the big picture show?*" They camped out in the library and looked and looked, but there was no answer. Incredibly, no one had done a systematic review of all of the evidence.

Beginning in 1984, with help from Stephanie Booth-Kewley and other graduate students, I embarked on a five-year attempt to fit everything together.

Meta-analysis

Almost all scientific studies in the life sciences end with the cautionary note, "Further research is needed. . . ." Conclusions are never final in science. The next study may show an unknown or unexpected qualification or exception to the previous conclusion. In fact, a book like this one may be criticized for going too far, because all of the data are not in yet. However, I believe that a lot more data are in already than most people realize.

The statement that further research is needed assumes that knowledge is cumulative. One study presumably builds on previous work. Is this necessarily the case?

Professor Robert Rosenthal of Harvard is well known for his study of the Pygmalion effect in the classroom. In this famous study, conducted two decades ago, Rosenthal found that children who were expected by their teachers to "bloom" intellectually did so. What was so interesting was that the teachers' expectations were based not on real evidence but on randomly created evidence—that is, teachers were given false information about which students had high IQs.

Not surprisingly, Rosenthal's study received a mixed reaction from the educational community. It suggested that teachers were unintentionally influencing their students. As applied to minority groups, it implied that minority children were failing in part because their teachers had low expectations for them. A storm of protest arose. Rosenthal, who is one of the nicest professors at Harvard, was bitterly attacked.

Fortunately, after the yelling and screaming is done, scientists usually return to their labs to try to prove the other guy wrong. And so hundreds of studies were conducted on the so-called expectancy effect (or Pygmalion effect, or Rosenthal effect). Many of these studies did find an effect, but some did not. How could the results be combined and viewed together?

To address these issues, Professor Rosenthal turned to *meta-analysis*, work that originally was developed by statisticians and then was updated by social scientists. Meta-analysis may sound philosophical and far-out, but it is really a fairly simple statistical technique for combining the results of studies.

Simply put, meta-analysis is a kind of average. Take, for example, a schoolteacher who gives a spelling test to her class and finds that the girls do 10 percent better than the boys. That is one "study." The school principal then gathers information on spelling from all of the classes in the school and finds out whether girls do better on average. This is what meta-analysis does; it combines the results of individual studies into an average.

Meta-analysis has several nice features. First, it forces the researchers to look at how *big* a relationship or effect really is. Many researchers are much too dependent on "statistical significance," which is probably the most widely misunderstood and misused concept in all of social research. With meta-analysis, the focus is on whether a finding is a strong one or a weak one.

Other benefits of meta-analysis pertain to increased attention both to the specific data and to patterns of findings. It is not enough to just read a study and walk away with a general impression of the findings. Meta-analysis forces examination of exactly what was done in a study and how strong the overall evidence is. By the way, Professor Rosenthal discovered that the Rosenthal effect is reliably found across hundreds of studies.

A similar situation exists regarding personality and health. There are many studies, but they use different methods and research designs and they have varying results. Could meta-analysis be used to make sense of all this? That is exactly what I did.

As a cautionary note, I should point out that meta-analysis can lead one astray if not thoughtfully conducted. For example, if ten bad (biased) studies are combined through meta-analysis, the outcome is one big biased result. Fortunately, our original meta-analyses and subsequent follow-ups showed some very striking patterns, even when various potential problems were taken into account.

Meta-analyses
of Personality and Health

What did we include in the first meta-analyses? Some of the most widespread speculation about health in the popular press concerns the effects of emotional states on arthritis and asthma. Other attention focuses on headaches and ulcers. Fortunately, there is also a reasonable amount of scientific research on these health problems, and we included them all. As a comparison, we also included coronary heart disease, for which, as we have seen, there is overwhelming evidence that psychosocial factors play a causal role.

In these systematic analyses, we examined every relevant study published between 1945 and the mid-1980s. Some of these studies contained interesting insights but could not be included in our statistical meta-analyses. For example, some of the research reports were only case studies in which a clinician reports that the patient's asthma seems to have come from emotional repression. Other studies did not include enough information in their published reports. Sometimes scientific journal editors, in their zeal to save space, ask authors (scientists) to cut down the length of their scientific manuscripts. There is usually a period of negotiation between the author and the editor (and with the journal's manuscript reviewers) to produce an acceptable article. All too often, information that may be useful to future investigators is dropped or condensed.

After reviewing all of the studies, we found over one hundred that could be included in the statistical meta-analyses. These studies in turn had assessed many thousands of people. We had arrayed before us almost all of the relevant published scientific work on the question

"Why are some people more likely to become ill?" As we calculated the relationships between disease and emotional aspects of personality, I could hardly wait to see the results.

Arthritis

Rheumatoid arthritis is an inflammatory disease of the joints that causes severe pain and disability. Eventually there is damage to the cartilage and bone. In Western societies, over 1 percent of the population suffers from arthritis; the elderly are especially vulnerable.

Traditionally, arthritis has been thought to be more likely to occur in people who are depressed or repressed, perfectionistic, and unable to express anger. Certainly it is true that people who suffer from arthritis are more likely to feel emotionally distraught, and various clinicians have argued that these feelings, in turn, tend to make things worse.

In our meta-analyses, we found that arthritis was clearly associated with depression, anxiety, hostility, and introversion. People with arthritis generally were more likely to suffer from emotional disturbances, especially anxiety and introversion but also hostility and depression.

One sixty-two-year-old arthritis sufferer we studied fit this pattern almost exactly. Sandra was a classic phlegmatic. She did not like her job on a production line, but she did not do anything about it. She did not like the town in which she was living, but she had lived there for seventeen years.

Sandra's voice was such a soft monotone that at times her speech was barely audible. She kept her arms folded in front of her chest. She reported that she would hold in anger when confronted and would never yell at an associate.

Sandra was always on time for her appointments and appeared quite neat, but she moved listlessly and spoke slowly. She was especially submissive when with people she did not know well. Her favorite hobbies were watching TV, going for drives, and gardening. When questioned, she denied any feelings of depression.

Does this repressed pattern make sense in terms of what we know about the biology of arthritis? The exact causes of arthritis are not fully understood, but the common types usually involve a problem with the body's immune system. For some reason, the body goes out of control and attacks some of its own cells. Given our current knowledge of the immune system, this physiological reaction seems like it would indeed be encouraged or even instigated in part by the emotional imbalance of repressed hostility or chronic anxiety.

Additional research is starting to fill in the precise physiological pieces of this puzzle. For example, one recent study made an intensive investigation of thirty-three women with rheumatoid arthritis. The researchers measured major challenges, minor daily hassles, and psychological distress among these women, then assessed the status of their immune systems through blood tests. Sure enough, this study found direct effects of stress on immune system functioning in these arthritic patients.

I cannot resist mentioning another study of arthritis that was conducted in the 1970s, titled "The Rheumatoid Personality: A Psychodiagnostic Myth." Contrary to what one may infer from the title, this study did not find that arthritis was unrelated to psychosocial disturbance. Instead, the study asserted that the arthritic personality was a myth because while people with arthritis differed from normal people, they looked similar psychologically to people with gastric ulcers, low back pain, and multiple sclerosis. In other words, these researchers concluded that there may be a more general, chronic disease-prone personality. Unfortunately, their insightful suggestion was lost in a sea of research findings.

Asthma

Bronchial asthma, characterized by wheezing and gasping for air, involves blockage of air exchange in the lungs. As it affects about 5 percent of the U.S. population, it is a major health problem. It is often disabling and sometimes fatal. Asthma rates have been rising steadily in the United States during the past decade.

All sorts of peculiar explanations for a link between emotions and asthma have been proposed. For example, one clinician's syllogism went as follows: (1) stimulation of anal and genital mucosae (mucous membranes) stimulates respiration; (2) stimulated and sensitized respiration promotes asthma; so therefore, (3) asthma may be caused by aggressive excretory fantasies that stimulate the genitals. Such speculations about the role of fantasy in asthma are nearly impossible to verify; carried to extremes, they caused the area of psychosomatic medicine to fall into disrepute in the 1960s.

Still, many asthmatics do report that their attacks are more likely to occur when they are under stress. One young female asthmatic we recently studied fit a typical pattern. Neat and pleasant, Mary seemed somehow overcontrolled and stressed. For example, when describing a happy summer vacation in Scotland, she sat still and did not look happy. An extensive battery of tests and measures revealed Mary to be extremely anxious. She felt weak and powerless, unable to control her life. Interestingly, she was, at the same time, a very angry and hostile person, ready to strike out at those around her. Many people with such a personality configuration are not asthmatic—they do not have the precise combination of individual characteristics, genetic makeup, and environmental challenges that leads to asthma's development—but it is not surprising to find an asthmatic with the above-described personality.

Our meta-analyses confirmed that asthma clearly is associated with anxiety and that asthmatics also are likely to be hostile or depressed. Although the exact causal role played by these negative emotions has not yet been uncovered, there are several plausible possibilities.

It now seems likely that asthma is first triggered by an allergen, such as pollen or dust, or by a lung infection. The bronchial mucosae swell, air intake is blocked, and the patient feels pain and terrible anxiety. The emotional reactions then make the asthma worse.

At that point, the body learns some very bad habits. Sometimes simply thinking about the allergy trigger ("the pollen count is going to be high today") can be enough to set off an attack. (This Pavlovian conditioning of allergic response has been demonstrated in laboratory rats.) The anxiety then compounds the physiological problems.

Furthermore, the attack may have some desirable social consequences, especially for children; they may receive sympathy and attention and be excused from school. Asthma attacks then become more frequent, and emotional disruptions intensify as the parents become more distraught. This vicious cycle is difficult to break.

The asthmatic patient, who probably was somewhat anxious or

hostile to begin with, then becomes more emotionally upset and is labeled a full-fledged asthmatic. The asthma is real and can be life-threatening. Sometimes parents recognize the vicious cycle and attempt to stop it by screaming something like "Stop your asthma attacks!" Unfortunately, it is much easier for the body to learn bad habits than to unlearn them. But as we shall see, a self-healing personality can be developed over time.

In short, a simplistic analysis that tries to ascertain whether anxiety "causes" asthma is inadequate. Anxious, powerless people do not necessarily develop asthma, and asthma is not "all in your head." However, certain maladaptive patterns of emotional response do indeed promote asthma attacks in susceptible individuals.

Headaches

Almost everyone has an occasional headache, but millions of people suffer from severe, disabling headaches. Muscle-tension headaches come from sustained contraction of the head and neck muscles. Often you can feel the "knot" in such a person's shoulders. The person's whole head hurts and may feel like it is in a vise. There is little doubt that chronically tense people are more prone to tension headaches.

Migraine headaches involve a blood vessel disorder in the vessels in the head. The vessels dilate and swell, and severe pain and nausea result. Many studies suggest that migraines can be brought on by stress, but what is the role of personality?

An interesting examination we did of a woman with weekly migraines found her to be highly anxious, depressed, insecure, somewhat introverted, but not at all hostile. She did not appear to be struggling with herself but rather appeared classically melancholic. She wanted to be happy, but something about her kept pushing her toward the distress. She told us that her father had been successfully cured of a brain tumor. Were her migraines some kind of psychic representation of a fear that she, too, would develop a brain tumor? I do not know, and I do not really think it matters. We never can be sure of such abstract interpretations, and understanding the abstract is generally not necessary for improving health. What is more important is the fact that this woman was not doing the things in her daily life that could make her more fulfilled and content.

Our meta-analyses found that headaches are associated with anxiety and depression. Surprisingly, though, we found very few decent studies of headaches and hostility. Although many theorists have proclaimed that headaches are caused by excessive anger, the matter has never really been adequately studied. However, it is clear that headache sufferers are not likely to be your basically happy, relaxed, and fulfilled individual.

Although the exact details of headache development have not been established, evidence strongly suggests that a general interruption in homeostasis is involved. The process often works as follows: First there is some disruption in normal physiological rhythms—an interference with sleep, a change in diet, a stressful change in daily routine, or even a sudden change in the weather. The hormonal and energy (metabolic) balances in the brain are disrupted, and the blood vessels may first constrict but then overdilate, causing pain. For example, if I get up too early in the morning, eat an inadequate breakfast, and rush off to sit in a hot airplane, I am sure to develop a terrible headache. If I regularly put myself in such situations, as my body learned to react in this pattern, I would become a chronic migraine sufferer.

Each person with headaches has certain individual imbalances that set off the headaches. Those people who head down the road of chronic anxiety and homeostatic disruption become regular headache sufferers.

Ulcers

Ulcers are sores in the lining of the stomach or upper part of the small intestine. They can cause severe pain and bleeding. As with heart disease, ulcers were rare until the last century or so.

In the mid-nineteenth century, Dr. William Beaumont treated a man whose stomach had an opening to the wall of his belly. He noticed that the secretion of stomach juices changed when his patient was emotionally stressed. Arguments about the role of stress in the development of ulcers have raged ever since. In fact, often I have seen the same arguments repeated and repeated in articles, with the recent authors having no idea that the matter is many, many years old.

It has long been thought that ulcers are more likely to occur in hard-driving people who worry too much, but in fact, the findings support the "worry" aspect, not the hard-driving part. There is good evidence that negative emotional states are related to a breakdown in the normal chemical balance between the protective stomach lining and the acid in the stomach. This is usually but not always an over-secretion of acid in response to stress. If rats are stressed, for example, they are more likely to develop ulcers. This fact was also well known by Dr. Hans Selye, who pointed out that epidemics of "air-raid ulcers" occurred in heavily bombed cities of Great Britain during the Second World War.

There are interesting historical differences between men and women in their ulcer rates. In western Europe in the late nineteenth century, young women had a much higher ulcer rate. In the twentieth century, the situation reversed; men became more likely to have ulcers. Such epidemiological differences strongly suggest that ulcers are heavily influenced by social and emotional, rather than purely biolog-ical, factors.

A particular point of contention has been over whether ulcers are influenced by a specific internal emotional conflict or by more general feelings of anxiety. What does the evidence show? Our meta-analyses, as well as other recent studies, found that ulcers are associated with chronic anxiety, depression, and an introverted personality. Unlike some chronic diseases, ulcers do not seem to be associated with a competitive hostility, but they definitely are related to having a weak personality in a challenging situation. So there is some truth to the notion that ulcers are more likely to occur in a melancholic or phleg-matic person than in a choleric or sanguine individual.

One ulcer patient we studied looked quite Type B on the surface. He was a government employee, friendly, thrifty, and physically fit. He was not at all competitive, but he liked to see things done right. Underneath, he was indeed a worrier. It was mostly the little things that bothered him. He was annoyed by litter, by sloppily made prod-ucts, and by the daily evidence of ethnic prejudice. He feared flying and large crowds. Everybody liked him, but he was not self-disclosing and had few close friends. He developed a terrible stomach ulcer.

Ulcers are not caused solely by emotional disturbances, but they are affected by emotional reactions. In people with weak stomachs and bad habits that damage the stomach lining (such as excessive coffee drinking), anxiety and introversion can be the final push that leads to ulcer formation.

The Overall Findings

The degree of consistency in the overall findings is remarkable. First, the magnitude of the relationships between chronic emotional disturbance and these diseases was similar for all of the diseases. Furthermore, the associations are similar in magnitude to those of other risk factors, such as diet and lack of exercise.

Second, the type of associations between personality and these various diseases form sensible patterns. They also are akin to those found for cardiovascular disease, for which there is much stronger evidence that personality plays a causal role. In other words, there is ample evidence for disease-prone personalities.

When some of my initial findings appeared in print, the public reaction was enormous. Front-page stories appeared in such places as the science news section of *The New York Times*, and my telephone rang off the hook. It seemed as if people intuitively knew that their health was being affected by their emotional reactions, and they wanted to hear about the details. The reaction also spurred my own further thinking and research on this topic. The more I looked, the more convinced I became.

FAILURES TO REPLICATE

The term *failure to replicate* sounds like a problem belonging to an endangered species. In fact, the term is used by scientists to indicate that one experimenter has not been able to replicate or reproduce the findings of another experimenter.

In physics and chemistry, attempts to replicate findings are relatively straightforward, since physical laws of nature do not change from day to day. In the social, behavioral, and life sciences, attempts to replicate usually are not exact, since the next study has to use a different sample of people (or patients or organisms) in a somewhat different environment. Still, the next study should try to capture the essential elements of the original research design.

There are various special problems in trying to replicate findings in the field of personality and health. Here is a partial listing:

- Many diseases take a long time to develop, so long-term studies are needed.
- People may change their emotional reactions over time, thus eliminating their risk.
- Psychological measures of personality often are weak or non-standard (and so may vary from study to study).
- Personality may not be a problem if the individuals under study have other things going for them, such as good exercise routines and good genes.

The point is simply that we have to look at overall patterns of findings and see if the evidence is convincing. I think it is.

Perhaps the biggest problem of replicating research linking personality to health emerged from my meta-analyses. The scientific jargon for this problem is "lack of statistical power." But the idea is an important one. It underlies much of the controversy about health risks.

Consider the fictional but realistic example of a state public health officer who wanted to see if bubonic plague had disappeared from his state. (Plague is still found in some parts of the United States.) He examined the detailed health records of two cities with a population of 50,000 and found no cases of the disease. But in his state, the disease is rare, appearing in only about 1 in 300,000 people per year. Through statistical chance, the health officer missed real cases of the disease.

A similar situation applies to personality and health. As we have seen, an unhealthy personality is neither necessary nor sufficient to cause disease. Disease is not necessarily caused or solely caused by unhealthy emotions. Some emotionally imbalanced people live long and healthy lives. It is only when the right measures are applied to large numbers of the right people in the right situations that the findings clearly emerge. The direct effects of personality on health are probably about the same size as many commonly known risk factors. Although the relationship is small in absolute terms, the public health implications of disease-prone personalities are enormous.

Furthermore, the various risk factors *combine* to produce synergistic effects on health that go beyond the simple effects of any single factor. For example, a middle-aged man who smokes, eats fatty foods, and is often stressed has a risk of heart disease that is much higher than one would expect if considering each risk factor separately.

PSYCHIATRIC DISORDER AND MORTALITY

If emotional disturbances like anxiety and depression are predictive of ill health in the general population, then we also should expect to see this relationship in the psychiatrically disturbed population. Are pathologically disturbed people also prone to physical disease? Not every study shows such an association, but enough studies show the expected link to encourage us in this line of thinking.

How can we tell if "psychiatric cases" are prone to ill health? There are two useful ways of studying this relationship. The first is to follow people who are quite ill already. The fact that they are already ill makes it likely that some additional observable illness or death will appear in a relatively short period of time. (If healthy but depressed twenty-year-olds were followed for a year, you might not see any illness whatsoever.) The second type of study involves following large numbers of people for many years. Let us consider a recent example of each.

A study at the Washington University School of Medicine in St. Louis examined fifty-two patients who were undergoing cardiac catheterization (a heart test) and were found to have coronary artery disease. A psychiatric interview was used to determine which of these patients were suffering from depression. Other medical data also were collected. The patients were then followed up one year later. The study found that the presence of major depression was the single best predictor of the occurrence of cardiac events, such as heart attack or death, during the coming year.

A study in Sterling County, Canada, followed over one thousand adult psychiatric patients suffering from serious depression or anxiety disorders. This study found that so-called affective (mood) disorder, especially depression, was associated with higher mortality. Some of this higher risk of death was due to suicide and accidents, although even some of these victims were likely in poor health. But affective disorder also led to a higher rate of cardiovascular disease.

In summarizing their conclusions, the authors of this Canadian mortality study noted that a depressed person may report feeling "half-dead." They aptly concluded that their "present report leads us to suggest that during the period of investigation, depression was likely to result either in being half-dead or dead."

DON'T BLAME THE VICTIM

As residents of Hiroshima and U.S. Army veterans involved in early weapons testing can tell you, exposure to high levels of radiation from a nuclear explosion makes it likely that you will develop leukemia or lymphoma. It doesn't much matter whether you are a jogger or what your personality is like.

If you breathe high levels of cigarette smoke or certain other pollutants, there is a good chance that you will develop lung cancer. If you are a fair-skinned person living in a southern climate and you suntan regularly, there is a very good chance (perhaps one in four) that you will develop skin cancer. If you are a woman whose mother and aunts and sisters developed breast cancer, there is a good chance that you will develop breast cancer.

In all of these cases, there is little about the victim's emotional responses that can prevent the cancer. Disease is influenced not only by psychological factors but also by the genes we are born with and the environment in which we live. In fact, most instances of disease are caused by a convergence of factors. As the case of the comic Gilda Radner recently demonstrated, it is a sad fact of life that some people contract cancer and die of it at a young age, regardless of personality or heroic struggle.

The social critic Susan Sontag has pointed out that tuberculosis used to be seen as caused by the character of the afflicted. Some saw TB as the result of a weak or romantic personality. That viewpoint changed dramatically when the TB-causing tubercle bacillus was discovered. Sontag argues that the same misperception currently is applied to cancer patients—they are unfairly blamed for causing their illness.

Our tendency to blame victims for their own illness is strong for two reasons. First of all, most of us have some concrete concerns about our own health and mortality. If this nice friend of ours can develop breast cancer, are we not also vulnerable? It is psychologically more appealing for us to assume that we are different—that our friend is somehow responsible for her own illness. That way, we distance and protect ourselves from feeling personally threatened. Or, put in religious terms, our friend must have been immoral to bring on this terrible scourge.

The second reason we tend to blame people for their own disease has to do with our desire for a predictable world. We like to believe that if we work hard and take care of ourselves, things will work out reasonably well. But illness arises suddenly and progresses unpredictably. Illness is terribly unfair and nonsensical. This is an ancient moral dilemma. It is no accident that the Book of Job begins as follows: "There was a man in the land of Utz, whose name was Job; and this man was perfect and upright and feared God and avoided evil." And yet, terrible calamities and diseases befall Job, one after another.

It is also the case that many people are very willing to accept blame for their illness. If you say to a cancer patient, "Many cancer patients have a feeling of chronic frustration in trying to accomplish what they want to in life," then most patients will reply, "Yes, that's true of me." In fact, various studies have shown that people are willing to accept almost any vague personality description that is authoritatively attributed to them, even if the description is randomly chosen. This has led to many case studies ridiculously being cited as proof of a link between personality and disease.

Thus there is always a danger that a casual reader will thumb through a book such as this one and conclude that people with disease have brought it on themselves. Aside from the inhumanity and lack of compassion for suffering people that this view entails, it may lead to further problems and suffering for the victim. That is, such an observer may feel inclined to withdraw financial or emotional support from a sick relative or friend.

On the other hand, it would be a disservice to both the healthy and the ill to pretend that they can have no effect whatsoever on their prognosis. It is a big problem that recently about half of Americans agreed with the statement "There is not much a person can do to prevent cancer." Healthy people can indeed help themselves stay healthy, and people who are sick can increase their chances of recovery. We must walk this fine line between blaming patients on the one hand and absolving them of any role in their health on the other.

Cancer and other stigmatized diseases are not punishment for past sins. And diseases like cancer certainly are not solely the fault of an unhealthy personality. But just as we know that there are healthful and unhealthful foods to eat and beverages to drink, so, too, are there healthy and unhealthy patterns of emotional responding.

FITTING IT ALL TOGETHER

The ancient Greeks knew that a bitter choleric person, a hopeless melancholic person, and an emotionless phlegmatic person were prone to disease. The ancient Greeks did not know, however, that these emotional imbalances were caused by a mismatch between an individual's internal resources and the challenges of the external environment, and they did not know how to correct emotional imbalances. They incorrectly blamed the "humors." They also did not know that invading microbes (bacteria and viruses), relations with other people, and genetic predispositions all function together to affect health. They had good intuition but little relevant science.

In modern times, doctors, scientists, and even the general public have tried in many different ways to link psychosocial variables to illness. "Oh, his cancer was probably caused by his sense of loss from the death of his mother when he was only six years old." "Her cervical cancer was caused by her feelings of despair when her husband suddenly walked out after ten years of marriage." "His heart attack was caused by his fights with his boss." Although occasionally true, I do not believe in such simple and clear associations.

I do not believe that a single event that happened many years earlier can be the sole cause of a particular illness that occurs today. However, I do believe that there is overwhelming evidence that unhealthy motivations can, in certain situations, produce the chronic emotional imbalances that predispose us to illness.

Emotions such as anger or sadness are not themselves harmful. On the contrary, the presence of real feelings shows that a person is alive and is addressing the world around him or her. The oft-heard commonsensical advice "Don't get angry, it's bad for your health" is simply wrong! It is only when these negative emotional states become chronic and severe—in other words, when the basic equilibrium is lost—that disease is likely to occur.

Many solid studies of the past two decades have found clear links between personality and cancer, heart disease, or other serious illness. My own statistical reanalyses of hundreds of studies, coupled with my own laboratory research and ongoing reanalyses, provide a special vantage point for viewing the many kinds of studies currently being published concerning psychology and health. An overall picture emerges. It is clear that there are disease-prone personalities.

It is less certain that specific disturbances (such as depression) are more likely to promote specific diseases (such as cancer), but this also may be true to some extent. That is, emotional imbalance in general creates physiological disturbances that increase the likelihood of illness in susceptible individuals. On top of these influences there seem to be some specific effects of certain emotional states. For example, chronic hostility is definitely a threat to overall health, and it seems to have a special association with cardiovascular disease; anxiety and depression are generally unhealthy but may be especially relevant to diseases involving problems with the immune system. But these special effects or links have not yet been clearly proven.

This chapter has focused almost solely on the ways personality affects ill health through disruptions in normal emotional functioning. These matters are the heart of this book. But remember that personality also influences health through impacts on smoking, eating, driving, muscle tension, exposure to violence, friendship patterns, cooperation with medical treatment, and many other behaviors. That is, hostile, depressed, and apathetic people tend to engage in behaviors that damage their health. When all of these influences are added together, personality's effect on health is truly astounding.

If there are such clear links between personality and disease, then it makes sense that there also should be strong links between certain personalities and health. Certain emotional response patterns should be able to lessen the likelihood of disease. The Greeks called these response patterns "sanguine." These healing personalities are discussed in the next chapter.

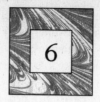

Personalities That Resist Disease: The Self-healing Personality

Bob Hope and Richard Pryor will go down in history as two of the twentieth century's great comedians. In addition to durable humor of wide appeal, their movies and shows are filled with intriguing social satire. Their performances also project very distinctive personal styles, and so most of us believe we have some knowledge of their personalities. Their contrasting public personas provide a good starting point for thinking about personalities that resist disease.

Hope's comedy projects a droll, bemused view of the world. Pryor's humor, in contrast, projects a suspicious and sometimes hostile view of the world. Both styles are clever and ironic, but, true to his name, Hope's style is the hopeful, auspicious, and sanguine one.

Which style is more likely to be a healthy one? Most people intuitively would feel that the cheerful, relaxed, low-key style of Bob Hope is healthier, even though Hope has worked hard his whole life and has faced many significant challenges. The scientific evidence indicates that his style would indeed be a healthy one for many people in modern society.

Is this true in all situations? Is there a situation in which the more aggressive and suspicious worldview may be healthier? Certainly in unpredictable or dangerous surroundings the suspicious approach is more adaptive, at least in the short run. It would allow the anticipation of problems. In other words, we should keep in mind the match between a person's orientation and the situations he or she faces. The difficulty, however, is that the aggressive and suspicious orientation often becomes injurious in the long run. It leads to unnecessary psychosocial disruptions, chronic negative emotions, and an increased likelihood of poor health.

There are daily threats to well-being; it is an achievement to stay healthy. Although this point may seem obvious when stated so simply, it is not the normal way we think about these matters. Instead, we generally assume that the normal state is to be healthy and that it is unusual to be ill. Thus we tend to overlook the psychological factors that promote a state of health.

Although most people know a thing or two about what constitutes a healthy life-style, their information is oversimplified and fragmented. If people understood the true nature of the self-healing personality, more changes would be forthcoming. Certain psychological characteristics promote the emotional states that function as part of a healing personality.

WHAT PHYSICIANS DON'T SAY

Although physicians are helpful to patients who are ill, they normally do relatively little to keep people healthy, especially in terms of psychological and social influences. Although there are important exceptions, the medical research establishment is similarly focused on a single issue: curing disease. This orientation has deflected proper attention from the question of health maintenance.

Each year, thousands of pages are published answering the question "Why did Ms. X become ill, and how can she be treated?" Little is asked about why Ms. Y remained healthy. Each week the prestigious *New England Journal of Medicine* publishes a "Case Record of the Massachusetts General Hospital," detailing the pathology of an unusual or informative patient's case. There is no corresponding "Case History of a Person Who Remained Well Throughout a Long Life."

The physician who does a fine job at implementing currently accepted medical treatments usually does not worry about individual differences among patients. For two fifty-year-old women with similar breast tumors and normal physiological stamina, the same treatment will be instituted; if one of them soon dies of her cancer, the treatment failure is attributed to "probabilities." Few physicians can be concerned about why two patients with similar conditions responded so differently to the same medical treatment.

One of my colleagues endured a terrible autumn. He developed a strep throat. His physician administered antibiotics and he was cured. A few weeks later, he again developed strep throat. More antibiotics. What happened? The same problem developed again. Finally the physician took throat cultures from the whole family. It turned out that my colleague's daughter was an asymptomatic carrier. That is, she had the strep bacteria and kept giving it to her father, but she had no symptoms of her own.

There are two important themes here. The first, of course, is that an understanding of health should take a person's environment into account. It makes no sense to keep treating the liver of an alcoholic who goes right back home to the booze. A truly successful health care provider must get out and examine the patient's situation, including the family and the work environment. Unfortunately, today's physician does not have the time, the training, or the resources for such activities.

The second lesson of the strep throat family comes from the daughter. Many people are exposed to bacteria (and other microorganisms) but do not get sick. This exact situation was documented many years ago in a study by two pediatricians. They followed a number of families for about a year, doing throat cultures for the strep bacteria every few weeks. What they found was that most of the strep infections did not produce any symptoms of illness! The strep bacteria by themselves could not cause illness. When the people were stressed, however, the strep illness was more likely to develop. On the other hand, of course, no one developed the strep illness without exposure to the bacteria.

Many people regularly encounter various environmental and physiological challenges and yet never seem to become ill. Others recover quickly, almost "miraculously," from serious illness. These observations have led to intriguing studies that seek to determine the personality structures that characterize individuals who remain healthy under challenge or who recover rapidly from illness. The self-healing personality is the subject of this chapter.

RATS AND CEOs

No, I am not trying to suggest that chief executive officers (CEOs) are rats. I did not invent the term *rat race*, used to describe the stresses of modern life. But many people take to the rat race analogy as accurately representing the dehumanized compulsion to get ahead in an unfeeling world. Fortunately for the analogy, resistance to disease has been studied extensively in both business executives and laboratory rats. I will begin with the nonhuman animals.

One of the most important series of studies of disease resistance concerns the development of ulcers in laboratory rats. The idea was that it would be unhealthy to lose control over one's environment—to be stressed and yet have no alternatives for action. To examine in detail the physiological effects of control, psychologist Jay Weiss placed his rats into one of several groups. Some of them heard a warning tone before receiving electric shocks.

The first rat was given electric shocks but could (and usually did) learn to exercise control in response to the preceding audible warning and thus avoid the shock. The second rat was "yoked" to the first rat; whatever happened to the first rat also happened to the second rat. In other words, the second rat had no control, but it would receive no more shocks than did the first rat. The results showed that the first group of rats, who could exercise some control over the shocks, developed much less ulceration than their helpless partners.

Other rats could (or could not) predict when the shocks were coming. Still other rats received no shocks. Of course, rats that did not receive any shocks showed the fewest health problems. Interestingly, though, the more predictable the threats, the healthier the rats remained.

There is a significant difference between the health of rats and the health of CEOs. Rats' responses are based on instincts and simple associative learning. Most executives have a cerebral cortex. Executives' responses depend more on thoughts and feelings, as influenced by their personalities.

A good human analogy to Dr. Weiss's rat studies concerns a small business in which there is a CEO, who makes the final decisions for the company, and a small advisory board of senior management personnel, who have a large investment of time and effort in the company. The most stressful situation for all is unexpected calamity, such as a major fire. But most threats develop more slowly. As threats to the company's survival appear, everyone on the management board sees the challenges and feels the stress; and the likelihood of illness rises for everyone. But only the CEO can easily apply control. Although the CEO has the greatest amount of work and responsibility, this position is *not* necessarily the most stressful. If the CEO has the best information, can exercise the most control, and has the right personality for the job, then health may be enhanced, rather than impaired, by the challenge.

The protective effects of controllable challenge are becoming better known. Even more important, however, are the individual strengths of the successful executive. About a decade ago, an extensive analysis of business executives under stress in a large midwestern firm examined the psychological differences between those who became ill and those who did not. Over a period of eight years, several key factors emerged.

First, as expected, the executives' feeling of control was significant. Those who remained healthier did not feel powerless in the face of external challenges but instead had a sense of power. Simply stated, they tended to believe that challenging situations could be influenced by their own efforts.

One of the executives studied, Andy, clearly lacked this sense of control. He appeared polite and eager to please, despite feeling increasing pressures of job responsibilities and job security. He carefully transmitted job orders from his superiors to his subordinates, but he exercised little authority himself. He worried that his workload was getting out of control. At home, trouble was developing with his wife and children. Andy had an ulcer and was on a restricted diet. He experienced sleeplessness, loss of appetite, and palpitations. Although only in his forties, he had a tendency toward high blood pressure. He lacked the strength of personality to cope with his job stress.

The second characteristic of executives who remained healthy was their commitment to something they felt was important and meaningful. Those individuals who felt committed to their work, the community, and their family were less likely to become ill. One executive, Bill, was seen as especially successful and healthy, even though his wife had been killed in an accident seven years earlier. He had a twinkle in his eye and a zest for his work. He enjoyed learning from his work, felt its social importance, and welcomed changes in the company as interesting and worthwhile.

Third, executives who did not become ill viewed life as a challenge rather than as a threat. They responded with excitement and energy. They were searching for novelty while remaining true to the fundamental life goals that they had already established. One of the successful, healthy executives, Chuck, was involved in difficult customer relations work. As his company began reorganizing, Chuck reported feeling more challenge but said it made his work that much more interesting and exciting. He did not feel threatened. Chuck was the kind of executive who views every problem as an opportunity to improve on the status quo.

This insightful research, by Dr. Salvatore Maddi and Dr. Suzanne Ouellette Kobasa, did much more than reveal specific characteristics that protect executives' health. It also provided a framework for thinking about staying healthy. Subsequent research, described later in this chapter, has further analyzed and described the personal characteristics that help a person remain well.

TWO STUDIES OF LAWYERS

Lawyers face many challenges in their work—the duties are by definition adversarial and the pace is fast. As part of a larger program of research, we happened to study two lawyers—one who was ill and one who was healthy. We found some suggestive differences. The ill lawyer, who was fighting heart disease, although pleasant on the surface, was extremely suspicious and almost became paranoid and combative about answering questions. The healthy attorney was very busy but exuded a sense of confidence and self-control. Interestingly, these impressions have been confirmed in two large studies of lawyers.

The first study involved 128 lawyers who initially were examined when they were in law school in the 1950s. At that time, they were administered a psychological test, which since has been refined into subscales measuring important aspects of the disease-prone personality. Of special interest were subscales that measured cynicism, hostile feelings, and aggressive tendencies—the choleric personality.

By 1985, thirteen of the lawyers (10 percent) in this study had died. As might be expected from population statistics, the deaths were due to heart disease, cancer, and diabetes. Was mortality related to personality? The results clearly showed that the higher one's choleric tendencies, the greater the risk of dying within the thirty-year period. In fact, the lawyers who scored at around the seventy-fifth percentile were about five times as likely to die as those who scored around the twenty-fifth percentile. Unfortunately, we do not know much about the social environments and the other behaviors of the lawyers during those thirty years.

The second study of lawyers looked at 157 lawyers in general practice. First the numbers of recent stressful challenges in their lives (such as hiring and firing staff members) were measured. Then the lawyers reported illnesses and symptoms experienced during the past year. Finally their personalities were assessed. Contrary to pop psychology theories, the happy-go-lucky, lackadaisical lawyers were not especially healthy. Common sense proved wrong again.

The healthiest lawyers were those who felt a greater sense of personal power and who were involved with and vigorously committed to their work. The healthy lawyers actively and positively addressed the challenges they faced; they did not become angry, apathetic, or depressed. These healthy lawyers also did not talk much to others about their work; it seemed as if professional demands and training precluded use of this usual means of maintaining psychological balance. Instead, they drew strength from their professional successes.

One lawyer I interviewed was an especially good example of this healthy style. Upon meeting him, one might never guess that he was an extremely hard worker, usually arising at 4:00 A.M. In his career, he made sure to keep a good mix of government and pro bono work. Much of it was challenging, but he always felt it was for a worthwhile purpose. He rarely talked about his work outside his office, since it could lead to quarrels with his friends; upon leaving work, he jogged to the train station to clear his head. Furthermore, knowing that he had phlegmatic tendencies, this lawyer made sure to spend evenings and weekends with his children and his warm and extroverted wife. He even joined the local PTA.

In short, given the special challenges of practicing law, certain personal characteristics are more protective against stress-related physiological imbalances. An aggressive, choleric manner is not healthy, but neither is a relaxed, laid-back style. Instead, active, involved lawyers with a positive motivation to do a good job are most likely to be healthy.

CONTROL

John Train is an investment advisor and insightful author who writes a monthly column in *Harvard Magazine*. Not long ago he wrote a profile of the investment advisor Philip Carret, who at the time was managing investment portfolios of $225 million. Carret arrived at his office on Forty-second Street in New York City early every morning—nothing remarkable until you realize that Carret was ninety-two years old. He had started money management in the 1920s! Here is how Train describes Carret: "He chuckles often; his personality radiates benevolence. When his stocks go down, Carret remains completely unruffled. Indeed, his friends do not detect any chink in his temperamental armor."

Mr. Carret or any investment advisor has, of course, very little control over his work world. Sometimes the unexpected and the terrible will occur. Ships can sink and stocks can crash. So how could he have such a healthy personality at age ninety-two? The answer is that it is not control over the world that is important to health. Dr. Weiss's rats revealed only part of the truth. Rather, it is a personal *feeling* of control, a sense that one can do as much as anyone can do.

A wild sense of optimism is not necessary for a healing personality. Instead, a sense that you can control your own behaviors is most important. Mr. Carret could gather all the financial information available and had complete discretion over which investments to make. In this sense, he was in complete control, even if the investments turned sour. This basic point is one of the most misunderstood in this area. It would be a gross oversimplification to assert that more control is better.

Thus, choice is important to health. A good example of loss of choice can arise when a worker is involuntarily laid off from work. One interesting study compared employed workers to workers who were laid off for long periods due to plant closings and who *remained* out of work. In terms of psychological states, the unemployed men had a lowered self-esteem and felt a loss of control. They felt they had nowhere to turn. In terms of emotional reaction patterns, the unemployed men were more depressed, anxious, angry, and irritable. These emotional states are in marked contrast to the investor, Mr. Carret, who "radiated benevolence."

In terms of physiological responses, the unemployed workers showed detrimental disturbances in blood pressure, cholesterol levels, blood sugar, and hormone levels. Rates of arthritis and ulcers increased. Although it is not clear exactly which states caused which reactions, it really does not matter that much, for it is clear that those workers with a high sense of control over their lives remained healthier, both mentally and physically.

Why is a sense of control so important? It seems that we have a basic motivation to gain a sense of mastery over our environment. Thirty years ago, Harvard psychologist Robert White called it a motivation toward *competence*. Most of us need to try to predict what will happen in our world. It is distressing and injurious to our health to have responsibility but no sense of control. A healthy work environment is one that provides a challenging, socially valued job and the resources and support with which to do the job. It does not matter if the job is sometimes very difficult.

Outside of prisons, it is hard to imagine a situation with less control than that faced by nursing home residents. They have no job, limited choices, and, sadly, little social value. Are these elderly residents doomed to deterioration and early death? A series of studies by Yale psychologist Judith Rodin has demonstrated that even minor interventions that increase the degree of control felt by nursing home patients can directly affect their health. Such interventions can be applied to almost all patients.

Control During Illness

"When I entered the hospital, I felt I was rapidly losing control of my life." These words can be found in any number of books by cancer patients. For people who are already seriously ill, many of the issues surrounding the healing personality come together in hospitals.

The word *hospital* derives from the same root as the word *hospitality*, but hospitals are not very hospitable places. Modern hospitals are organized with two goals in mind. The first is to bring together in one place all of the equipment and personnel—diagnostic equipment, life-support equipment, treatment equipment, physicians, nurses, technicians—to assist a body that has lost the ability to heal itself. The second goal is to avoid wasting the doctors' time. Whether there is a shortage or a surplus of physicians, the best way to provoke a physician into a furious rage is to leave him or her standing in a hospital room waiting for a missing piece of equipment.

In hospitals, patients lose control over what and when they eat, what they wear, when they sleep, and whom they can see. They have little say about who can touch them or when they can receive pain-control medication. Some of these losses are necessitated by the demands of their disease, but most are not. Although near-miraculous treatments sometimes take place in hospitals, and although the staffs are dedicated and hardworking, hospitals are not very healthy places from a psychological point of view.

For melancholics, who are becoming sadder and sadder about their illness, the loss of control in hospitals only makes matters worse. Depression is common. Phlegmatics, who are holding back their fears and anxieties, face hurried physicians and nurses and a general lack of privacy; it is not an atmosphere conducive to dealing with inner emotions. For cholerics, any anger or dominance vented in hospitals is likely to bring them trouble from the hospital staff, who may view them as troublemakers. Ironically, cholerics may then be even more restricted in their activities.

Radical changes should be wrought in hospitals; some reforms already are being made in response to pressures from social scientists. The best example of change concerns labor and delivery. Not all that long ago, a woman in labor was isolated from her husband, confined to bed, and, possibly, heavily anesthetized. The newborn was removed to a glass-enclosed nursery, away from the parents. Visiting hours for other family members were severely restrictive. All of this was thought to be in the best medical interest of the mother and the baby. Instead, it was simple prejudice. Today many women can have their babies in a homey hospital birthing room; families can be present and they can feel comfortable and at home. Even though high-tech medical interventions are available for emergencies, the women are able to feel more in control.

Regular hospital rooms and procedures should be similarly altered. In some cases, patients need special treatment or protection that necessitates extraordinary confinement. But in most cases, patients could have more control over what they wear, when and what they eat, who visits, and when they will sleep. Hospital staff needing to enter the room could introduce themselves and explain what they need to do. And so on. The result would be healthier patients and self-fulfilled staff. This is not to minimize the suffering and the life-and-death procedures that go on in hospitals. But a proper psychosocial climate would enhance, rather than interfere with, the usual medical treatment.

Some hospitalized patients assert their sense of control in their own ways. Let me give some examples. One patient constantly questioned his doctors and nurses. Another patient insisted on getting up and walking around his room immediately after surgery. A third patient covered the walls with greeting cards and telephoned all of her friends. Another had his wife bring in salami sandwiches. *These actions are good signs that the patient is endeavoring to regain emotional balance and have the self-healing processes work their best.* Such actions are characteristic of the self-healing personality, and they are recognized as such and encouraged by the wisest physicians.

Other patients develop a somewhat odd type of perceived control. They have learned to give up decision making to their caretakers when ill—at first their parents and now their doctors. Some do quite well for a while by insisting, "Whatever you say, Doc." Again the sense of choice is relevant—they have voluntarily given up power to the physician. In general, though, this strategy is less flexible in the long run.

One interesting recent study examined patients' degree of dispositional optimism on the day before they had coronary bypass surgery. The results of the study revealed that the optimists had a faster rate of recovery from the surgery. Furthermore, the optimists reached certain recovery milestones (such as walking around their rooms) sooner. But it is not optimism that promotes health. *Realistic optimism coupled with a plan for success* is more important for most people than is blind faith.

In sum, for most people, a sense or feeling that they are in control is healthy. For some people, the feeling that someone else is temporarily taking care of them can be healthy, especially if they cannot realistically be expected to exert control themselves. A person with a serious illness who is facing an operation needs to feel confident that the surgeons, nurses, and family members will do a good job; we should not force control onto people who do not want it. But as the patient's condition improves, he or she should regain some sense of competence. In general, the more people feel self-confident and in control of their lives, the healthier they will be.

COMMITMENT

In 1978, Anatoly (now Natan) Scharansky was convicted of treason in Moscow and was sentenced to many years at hard labor. His real crime was that he was a Jewish activist who was trying to emigrate to Israel. At the end of his trial, whose outcome had been predetermined, Scharansky stood up in court and addressed the following remarks to the observers: "Five years ago, I submitted my application for exit to Israel. Now I'm further than ever from my dream. It would seem to be cause for regret. But it is absolutely otherwise. I am happy. I am happy that I lived honestly, in peace with my conscience."

Scharansky survived many years in a Soviet prison and eventually was permitted to emigrate, in good health. While waiting, he did what he could, with help from his wife Avital, to advance his cause.

Although few Westerners face the challenges Scharansky faced, almost everyone is subject to environmental pressures. Yet many hard workers thrive anyway. Exactly opposite of what writers about workaholism and the Type A personality often claim, living life to the fullest seems to provide protection from disease. Sometimes the pace is hectic.

A key element of this healthy style, however, involves a commitment to an ideal greater than oneself.

Mohandas K. Gandhi (also called Mahatma, or "Great Soul") was one of the greatest workaholics of all time. He was not sickly, although he spent over twenty-three hundred days in prison and endured numerous self-imposed fasts. On the contrary, he had the personal strength and commitment to be one of the most influential leaders of the twentieth century, and perhaps of all time. He pioneered nonviolent political resistance (*satyagraha*), instituted numerous social reforms, and won political freedom for India. He was assassinated in his seventy-eighth year.

What defined Gandhi's life was a commitment to principle. As he aged, he grew more and more content with his life, but he remained humble. He certainly was not blindly optimistic, carefree, or lackadaisical.

Alienation is unhealthy. Obligation and dedication are healthy. Some people find this commitment in religion, others in philosophy. Other people seek political reform. Some people simply have a hobby, such as preserving old cars or old trees or old books. What they have in common is a sense of purpose.

The Japanese culture is known for fostering commitment to hard work in general and to one's company in particular. This commitment is healthy up to a point; it also can be carried to an unhealthy extreme. Many competitive Japanese are working longer and longer hours, with a consuming passion. The result? Japanese workers are now concerned about *pokkuri byo*, or sudden death, and *karoshi*, death from overwork. With little effort spent on anything but work, the workers lose their equilibrium. Emotional reaction patterns change from pride and contentment to distress and fatigue, and general homeostasis begins to break down.

CHALLENGE

Almost a decade ago, I was visiting Boston and wandered by the box office of a downtown theater. Luck was with me—excellent seats had been released just that minute for the next night's performance of Yul

Brynner in *The King and I*. The performance was outstanding, and Brynner received a long standing ovation.

I did not know it then, but Yul Brynner had cancer. When first diagnosed with a deadly carcinoma, he underwent massive radiation treatment, all the while performing in *The King and I*. He was determined to fight the disease while maintaining his quality of life. He had grown up with an attitude that said a person had to make the most of each day. Now, while in crisis, he relied on the ways of coping that he knew best. When doctors advised him to take it easy, he responded that he would remain active. More than a year later, when most patients with his condition would have been dead, he was performing to sellout crowds on Broadway.

Mr. Brynner's theater performances while fighting cancer, like Mr. Scharansky's travails in the Soviet Union, must have been extremely stressful, but they were never boring. *Boredom puts one at higher risk for disease. People who are constructively challenged find it easier to remain healthy.*

Many health promotion efforts do not appreciate this fact. Middle-aged cholerics are advised to slow down, retire, take it easy, rest. Starting down this path may lead them to dwindle and subside right into a rest home. On the other hand, melancholics do not need to be told to perk up. Rather, they need a *reason* to perk up—a challenge in their lives. Phlegmatics, too, need the energy and feelings of excitement that result from challenge.

The runner Mary Decker Slaney, who broke four world records, has faced many extreme stresses of competition. Yet she has stayed healthy and keeps competing. When asked why she runs, she answered, "I love it. Running is something I do for myself more than anything else." This is the healthiest view of challenge—something that brings positive emotions and a sense of personal triumph.

Boredom is a warning sign that health problems may be on the way. The German philosopher Arthur Schopenhauer said that the two foes of human happiness are pain and boredom. Self-healing personalities take risks appropriate to their personal strengths and individual situations. A middle-aged accountant did not need to take up skydiving; he did quite well starting his own new consulting business. But another man, tired of his insurance business and flabby in the belly, needed the high stimulation of learning to water-ski.

Emotional Training

When an athlete begins training, there is a period of struggle, weakness, and pain. A runner or water-skier will have sore legs, a weight lifter will have sore arms, and they will all feel fatigue. Soon, however, their muscles will enlarge and they will be stronger and more proficient performers.

A similar situation occurs as our bodies fight an infection or other disease. Certain physiological systems weaken, while others go into an emergency response mode. As the disease is slowly conquered, however, the systems return to a homeostatic state, often stronger than ever.

Not surprisingly, an analogous sort of training occurs in the self-healing personality. Emotional balance also can become "fit" and "hardy." Individuals who seek out moderate emotional challenge initially may feel weak and discouraged, they are fatigued, and they feel emotional pain. But this pain or struggle in the short run enhances their emotional stability in the long run. Contrary to the simplistic advice to avoid stress, the experience of moderate challenge can help condition healthy emotional responses.

Physiological research supports this view. "Arousal reduction" is not necessarily healthy. Rather, a kind of physiological toughness can develop in competitors that serves to buffer the effects of future struggles. This is especially true for playful, expressive, challenge-seeking individuals.

The case of a forty-one-year-old heart attack victim we interviewed provides a good example of training in progress. When asked how he felt about waiting in lines, such as bank and post office lines, this tense, competitive man interjected loudly, "I don't like waiting in lines." But he explained that he now would choose the longest line at K mart so that he could practice "not letting it bother me." This individual also was learning how to spend time with his two young sons, even when they acted childish. Fortunately or unfortunately, he now had plenty of time to spend with them, since his heart attack had forced him to retire from his job. (Various techniques for self-improvement are described in chapter 8.)

Dr. Walter Cannon, who developed the idea of homeostasis, emphasized that the body has developed a margin of safety. By this Cannon meant that the body is not built with "niggardly economy" but rather has some allowance for contingencies that we may count on in times of stress. The lungs, the blood, and the muscles have much greater capacity than is ordinarily needed. The liver, pancreas, stomach, and other digestive and metabolic centers can be seriously damaged and yet still sustain life. And so on. In other words, the body naturally prepares itself for the rare "extra" challenge, and so it is natural and prudent to do what we can to increase these margins of safety.

The turn-of-the-century philosopher and psychologist William James, who anticipated much of our modern scientific understanding of emotional responses, summed up this idea succinctly when he advised:

> Keep the faculty of effort alive in you by a little gratuitous exercise every day. That is, be systematically ascetic or heroic in little unnecessary points, do every day or two something for no other reason than that you would rather not do it, so that when the hour of dire need draws nigh, it may find you not unnerved and untrained to stand the test.

HEALTHY SUBTYPES

Thomas is a very hardworking executive with all sorts of additional responsibilities to his community. He is married with four children, and he always seems to be on the run. Yet he is the picture of health. He has many friendly colleagues and is easily approachable because of his sense of humor. He takes no drugs and drinks only on occasion. He takes a month's vacation with his family every August and another weeklong vacation in the winter. He associates often with an extended circle of friends from his same ethnic (Latin) background. He enjoys parties.

Sean is a middle-level manager with an intellectual bent. He speaks softly but clearly and firmly. He likes to read and to travel with his wife. He has tried his hand at writing fiction and belongs to a small writers' group. He jogs and lifts weights. He has no health problems.

Self-healing personalities have an inherent resilience, but they are not identical. They share an emotional equilibrium that comes from doing the right combination of activities appropriate for the individual.

It is useful to think about two major types of self-healing personalities. The first is the more active, gung-ho type. This includes the busy but confident lawyer, and the hardworking executive, Thomas. These people actively seek out stimulation, are highly extroverted, and tend to be spontaneous and fun-loving.

The second main type of self-healing personality is more calm and relaxed. In American society, it is the image projected by Bob Hope—active, alert, involved, and responsive, but calm, philosophical, and bemused. This is the serenity, or *galenos*, of Galen. Although these people also enjoy the presence of others, they are more likely to have a few close friends than dozens of partygoing acquaintances.

These two types of healthy people have different optimal levels of stress. For the second, more reserved and content type of person, it is better to have conflicts resolved and stimulation under control. For the first, more excitement-seeking type of healing personality, a higher level of challenge is healthier. Unsolved dilemmas are not a bother.

In line with this way of thinking, research suggests that in similar situations, these two types of people have different tendencies toward negative emotions and stress hormones. The low-key, goal-oriented individual shows more distress and has a greater release of stress hormones when challenges remain unresolved. The more spontaneous and arousal-seeking individual, on the other hand, is especially likely to be distressed by a lack of stimulation and feels threatened only when challenges become too much to handle. Thus, here again we see that blanket health recommendations for the whole population can lead to serious problems. The individual must be considered.

How can these two main types of self-healing individuals be identified? The easiest way is to observe them in social activities and see how they respond—as droll and bemused or active and fun-loving. Another way is to use questionnaires. Low-key, goal-oriented individuals tend to agree with statements like "I plan ahead," "I prefer interesting but safe courses of action," and "My laugh is soft and subdued, but I chuckle often." The more spontaneous and arousal-seeking individual, on the other hand, tends to agree with statements like "I enjoy taking risks," "I would make a good actor," "I enjoy parties," and "I hug my friends when the mood moves me."

THE WILL TO LIVE, AND THE WILL TO DIE

Several years ago, an incredible story about Felipe Garza was reported throughout the media. Felipe was a fifteen-year-old boy, living in California, who fell in love with a fourteen-year-old named Donna. With echoes of Romeo and Juliet, it soon developed that Donna was dying of degenerative heart disease. Felipe, who seemed in fine health himself, went to his mother and told her that when he died, he wanted Donna to have his heart.

Less than a month later, Felipe suffered a cerebral hemorrhage—a burst blood vessel in his brain—and he died. As he had requested, his heart was transplanted to his girlfriend Donna by surgeons in San Francisco.

Except for some investigation of cases of voodoo death, no one has much studied the concept of a will to die. It certainly does not seem likely that a teenager could will himself a stroke. Yet for every single disease that I have reviewed in the medical literature, there are at least some cases in which a primary contributing cause of death was said to be a psychological will to die. Puzzling cases like Felipe Garza are useful in stretching our thinking on this issue. It is plausible that we are *underestimating* the powers of self-healing.

Although we hear little about healthy people developing a will to die, the idea of a will to live is common both in popular culture and in medical circles. All sorts of pop health books describe case after case of patients who hear some bad news, show some far-off look in their eyes, lose the will to live, and quickly succumb; these cases are compared to individuals who supposedly make up their minds that they will beat their illness. Unfortunately, the will to live is often viewed as some mysterious, unfathomable force.

The will to die involves the disruption of a physiological process to such an extent that it cannot be restored—a passage beyond the point of no return. But the will to live involves growth. It concerns the stimulation of complementary physiological processes that correct the disturbance. It is interesting to note that there is no middle ground—stagnation is unhealthy. Body processes are dynamic and always active. If you are not living, then you are dying.

In 1985, seventeen-year-old unseeded Boris Becker defeated Kevin Curren to become the men's singles champion in tennis at Wimbledon. A turning point came early as Becker broke Curren's serve, and Curren never had the confidence to regain his most powerful weapon. As the match wore on, Becker gained in determination while Curren saw his willpower wane.

Most people will accept this description of a sports match without any qualms. It is clear that intangible "willpower" can affect the outcome. The same kinds of intangibles can affect health. Some people have a greater will to live.

For several decades earlier in this century, Harry Hoxsey, a former coal miner, sold a "successful" cure for cancer. Hoxsey's clinics spread to seventeen states as patients testified as to the miraculous cures brought on by his potions. Hoxsey's cure for cancer worked for some people because it stimulated their bodies' own self-healing systems. The Hoxsey potion was an extraordinary placebo. Unfortunately for Mr. Hoxsey, it did not work for him—he himself succumbed to cancer.

Almost everyone has heard about placebo effects, but few people understand their nature or power. Simply stated, a placebo is any intervention that does not have a specific, expected physiological effect on the body. For example, a sugar pill may be compared to a morphine extract for pain control; the sugar does not have any direct pharmacological action on the nervous system. So any effects of the sugar pill on pain are placebo effects. But they can be very real effects.

Placebos do not have to be sugar pills. They can be diets, exercise regimens, consultations with doctors, or any other procedures that may be encountered by patients, even by patients taking a pharmacologically active drug. We always need to look for placebo effects in order to see whether any patient reactions are due to the "real" drug or due to these other influences.

In the better medical journals, new treatments are always evaluated in comparison to a placebo control group. For example, to what extent did chest pain decrease or did joint mobility increase in the medication group as compared to the placebo group? Interestingly, the placebo group itself almost always improves, too (compared to baseline). Occasionally, the change due to the placebo is greater than that due to the drug. But often these placebo effects are ignored; they are seen as random variation or bias instead of as an important phenomenon in themselves.

Wise doctors know that a new drug almost always performs better when it is still new. Over time, as failures, limitations, and side effects become more apparent, the excitement and positive expectations surrounding the new treatment wane and the drug becomes less efficacious. Why not capture this positive influence and put it to use? Unfortunately, self-healing emotions cannot be distilled and put into a bottle. But they can be induced by encouraging individual patients to enter the psychosocial environments that are best for their health.

Contrary to what many believe, placebos, such as inert sugar pills, do have physiological effects. They can immediately cause nausea, rashes, diarrhea, fainting, pain, and drowsiness. Other effects may follow. Placebos also have been shown to promote healing of wounds, recovery from surgery, the elimination of pain, and the reduction of fever. Their effects seem to occur in two ways—through restoration of emotional imbalances and through encouragement of healthy behaviors. To take a simple but important example, a placebo pill can help a migraine sufferer if it relaxes the patient enough so that blood vessel dilation returns to normal levels, neck and head muscles unknot, appetite returns, and a refreshing nap can be taken. The placebo does not have any direct physiological effects on the nerves affecting the blood vessels, but its curative effects are no less real. Effects that do not occur in a test tube (in vitro) may well occur in vivo—in the complex system of the human body.

Not everyone is affected by placebos. Some estimates are that about one-third of patients are so influenced. Who are these patients? All of the evidence is not in yet, but it seems likely that they are the patients who are provided with the means to redress some emotional instability. For example, they may be depressed people who need some hope, hostile people who need to channel their energies in a productive direction, or repressed sufferers who are given a way to get in touch with their inner selves.

When people "find their niche" or "hit their stride," the balance and harmonic rhythms of their daily living lead to ongoing positive emotions. It is these positive emotions that are associated with the beneficial physiological changes that may result from placebos.

Will-to-Live Emotions

In emotional terms, I like to think of the sanguine, self-healing personality in terms of "enthusiasm." The word *enthusiasm* literally means "having a godly spirit within." "Cheerfulness" is another good emotional term. Deriving from the word for *face, cheer* at one time referred to facial expression. Cheerful people express good spirits through their faces.

Enthusiastic people are successful in accomplishing tasks and helping others. They are alert, responsive, and energetic, although they also may be calm and self-assured. They are curious, secure, and constructive. The emotional aspects of their personality are apparent to the trained observer.

I have been studying the nonverbal emotional style of the self-healing personality for many years. There are several good clues that indicate emotional balance and an inherent resilience.

Enthusiastic, sanguine people tend to infect others with their exuberance. They are not ecstatic but rather they are generally responsive and content. They are people you like to be around.

Good eye contact is one easily observable sign. Sanguine people look you in the eye during a greeting and a substantial portion of the time while talking and listening. They are not downcast or shifty-eyed. Sanguines also smile naturally—the eyes, eyebrows, and mouth are synchronized and unforced; there is usually no holding back of expression of pleasant feelings.

Sanguines have smooth gestures that tend to move away from the body. (That is, they are less likely to pick at, scratch, and touch their bodies.) They are unlikely to fidget, and their legs are often uncrossed and open rather than tight and defensive. They are not apt to make aggressive gestures with their hands.

Emotionally balanced individuals not only walk smoothly, they talk smoothly. They are inclined to show fewer speech disturbances, such as saying "ah," and their speech is modulated rather than full of sudden, loud words. Sanguines' voices are less likely to change in tone when under stress.

Obviously, there are exceptions to these rules. A single nonverbal gesture does not reveal much. Still, it is remarkable how much valid information we can gather about a person's healthy emotional style from just a few episodes of social interaction.

CREATIVITY AND PLAY

It is not coincidence that performers like Katharine Hepburn, Vladimir Horowitz, and Pablo Casals, who remained successful late in life, also retained that magical spark and joie de vivre that audiences find so appealing. The joy, fulfillment, and playfulness of living are key aspects of the self-healing personality.

The influential psychologist Carl Rogers was the first to call scientific attention to personal growth and fulfillment—the joy of being alive. Rogers saw each person as having an inherent tendency to grow and enhance his or her being—discovering a true self that may be hidden—in order to produce more positive inner feelings. The fully functioning person lives up to his or her potential and completely develops and uses any talents.

Rogers primarily was concerned with psychological health, but it turns out that he described a basic component of general health. This is not so surprising, since the many patients Rogers saw in therapy were facing major emotional imbalances. Rogerian therapy involves helping patients to clarify their feelings so that they can integrate their unique life experiences into their self-concept, thus releasing their inner creativity.

For example, one male heart attack victim we studied was a very hard worker at work but did little but lie on the couch at home. He was not satisfied with his job level, and he would have preferred to live in a more easygoing environment. For him, the beginning of the road to recovery came in his recognizing that he was in the wrong line of work and really should be pursuing his love of the outdoors. Once this insight was achieved, his other problems began to resolve. This line of thinking further supports the idea that a healing personality is some-what different for each individual.

Rose Fitzgerald Kennedy, the mother of President John F. Kennedy, faced many severe challenges in her life, including the disability and death of her husband and the deaths of four children. Yet she has lived an exceptionally long, productive life. Now a hundred years old, she emphasizes the importance of growing and learning, of vivacity, curiosity, and true interest in other people. In her book *Times to Remember*, she sums up her philosophy by saying that optimism feeds on itself. "I'm sure God wants us to be happy and take pleasure in life," she concludes.

Mrs. Kennedy certainly is not always happy. Neither are most self-fulfilled artists and performers. In fact, they are often quite moody. But if their inner creativity can be harnessed and ridden toward the exploration of new personal heights, a psychological and physical glow of good health emerges. It is the glow of a joyful, peaceful emotional harmony.

I do not wish to sound theological or metaphysical here. Creativity and spontaneous play do not have to be conceived of as inexplicable divine genius. Rather, there are identifiable thoughts and behaviors that characterize creative and self-fulfilled individuals.

The humanistic psychologist Abraham Maslow spent a good part of his influential career focused on the positive, growth-oriented aspects of human beings. Dr. Maslow recognized that healthy people first need to achieve balance in their basic biological needs, and then they need to obtain affection and self-respect. But he emphasized "self-actualization"—the realization of personal growth and fulfillment. People with this growth orientation are spontaneous and creative, are good problem solvers, have close relationships with others, and have a playful sense of humor.

As people become more self-actualized, they become more concerned with issues of beauty, justice, and understanding. They develop a sense of humor that is philosophical rather than hostile. They become more independent and march to the beat of a different drummer. They become more ethical and more concerned with harmony among members of the human race. These characteristics of the self-healing personality are not merely the opposite of such disease-prone characteristics as suspiciousness, bitter cynicism, despair and depression, or repression of conflicts. Rather, they are positive, meaningful motives, behaviors, and goals in their own right.

Talking to victims of serious illness, it is intriguing to note the ways many of them have changed their philosophies of life after their brush with death. A reasonable expectation is that recognition of the fragility of life may lead to a callous and hedonistic rampage—"I might as well maximize my fun, because I won't live forever." In fact, such reactions are rare. For people who make changes (many do not), the direction is almost always toward greater self-fulfillment. Here are some representative comments:

"I try to spend more time with my family."
"I stop to smell the roses."
"I try to see the other guy's side of things."
"I spend more time reading."
"I do volunteer work at the hospital."
"I've taken up painting."

Ironically, many of the illnesses could have been postponed or avoided if these people had made such changes earlier in their lives.

I said earlier that self-healing emotions cannot be put into a bottle. This is true, but I predict that someone will try. Given the tremendous power of the traditional medical approach to disease, I can make the following forecast with confidence: As the healing powers of emotional balance become more and more apparent, some biochemist will try to isolate the most important hormones and other chemicals that the body releases in restoring homeostasis—with the goal of bottling and selling homeostasis healing pills.

SOCIAL TIES AND SOCIAL INTEGRATION

One reason that a solely biological approach to health is miserably inadequate is that people are social beings. We are born into families, are raised in communities, and live in societies. All sorts of evidence indicates that major psychological and physiological abnormalities result when a child is raised without sufficient, high-quality human contact.

The basic elements of a self-healing personality develop during childhood. Although this has long been recognized, early psychoanalysts focused on the internal conflicts and frustrations of childhood. The attention was generally on the negative aspects of human nature—on what could go wrong. Dr. Erik Erikson, on the other hand, turned the Freudian framework on its head. He showed that human struggles can be seen in terms of the positive and successful resolution of tensions, especially in regard to social relations.

Dr. Erikson underscored the idea that although stressed children could come to feel mistrustful, guilty, and inferior, they could instead become trusting, autonomous, and industrious. In adulthood, the individual may succumb to identity crises, isolation, stagnation, and despair; but many people triumph over life's challenges and develop self-esteem, intimacy, altruism, and existential satisfaction. Throughout life, the healthy personality continually develops what is best in himself or herself, while also helping others to thrive.

At the risk of oversimplification, healthy psychosocial development can be summarized in terms of one basic ongoing process—disclosing one's feelings to loving others. For young children, this means expressing joy or despair and having a responsive adult there to understand. For older children, the process is one of trying (or playing) out different roles and having an emerging positive sense of self confirmed by the family. For adults, self-disclosure is key to developing intimacy and empathy with a spouse and close friends. For the elderly, the sharing of feelings with loving others strengthens the sense of life's meaning and the continuity of the generations. This is why self-absorption can be so unhealthy. Health resides not within an individual but within a social context.

The Family

When a person develops a serious illness like cancer, it is really the whole family that must fight the cancer; the stress affects everyone. However, medical treatment typically pays little heed to the family's needs. One physician, when he discovered that I dealt with the emotional side of health and illness, told me, "I think it's great that there are people like you who can keep the family members out of my hair so that I can get on with treating my patient." He was a good physician, but he had neither the training nor the inclination to deal with the social context of his patient's illness.

As we have seen, hospitalized patients routinely are cut off from their families and friends. When the patient then returns home and reintegrates into the community, the medical system does not follow along to ease the way and monitor recovery. When physicians stopped making house calls, they thought they were becoming more efficient and effective. In many cases they were. But becoming cut off from the patient's home environment leaves the physician ignorant about how best to treat each patient's unique needs. This is why physicians who do venture out of their protected and regimented office suites are often greeted with such adulation by their patients.

Can these breaks with the family be repaired? In some instances they already have been remedied. Many towns now have hospices for terminally ill patients. The hospice may be a small clinic or may be based in the patient's home, but the common goal is to ease the transition to death. Most people familiar with hospices think of them as providing the pain relief and emotional support desperately needed by the terminally ill. They do indeed provide this. But hospices also "treat" the family. The emphasis is on emotional peace in a time of crisis. In fact, part of hospice treatment involves counseling the family after the patient has died.

The hospice is one example of how the family can be brought back into its rightful place in fighting illness. But other changes are possible, too. Example: Some pediatric hospitals make it comfortable for a parent to spend the night with an ill child. (This was almost unheard of a generation ago.) Why not make similar arrangements for spouses or friends of adult patients? Example: In most treatments, the patient cannot be accompanied by family members. This could be changed; many family members have proved to be valuable medical assistants. Example: It is rare for the patient, the family, the physician, and a social worker to sit down together and discuss the patient's illness and its effects on the family. But a few such discussions probably could prevent many health problems.

With these examples, I am offering some possible new directions to promote self-healing. They may not always be feasible, but I think they are worth considering in some detail. They are being used already by physicians and patients who have an intuitive sense of what self-healing is all about.

The Community

More than a decade ago, men and women living in Alameda County, California, were asked about their amount of contact with friends, relatives, and community groups. They were followed for nine years. The extent of social ties was strongly associated with the likelihood of staying alive. A large follow-up study was conducted on data collected in Finland. This study confirmed the protective effect of social ties, especially for men.

There are all sorts of studies indicating that people with closer community ties have better health habits, better mental adjustment, and better physical health. In dealing with challenge, these people have better sources of information, more help, and more advice. Most important, they have people they care about and who care about them. It is unhealthy to be lonely.

The Society

In Japan, the individual is seen as part of the whole. The individual works for the betterment of his or her family, company, and country. There is a high degree of loyalty, conformity, uniformity, and stability. The individual Japanese is highly integrated into society.

In America, there is relatively more independence. People change spouses, companies, professions, residences, and political loyalties with frequency. The social milieu is more independent, self-reliant, and alienating.

Which of these environments is healthier? All other things being equal, the more stable, uniform environment is healthier; it provides identity and meaning for the individual. However, other factors enter the equation. First, societies are not static. As technologies change, economies change, and politics change, the population must adapt. A rigid, structured society may make these adaptations more difficult for its population. Second, uniform, structured societies can become stultifying; such boredom and rigidity is unhealthy. Third, even in a uniform, stable society, influences from other cultures become known and create special problems for those to whom they appeal. For instance, it is more stressful to be a rock and roller or an investigative reporter in Japan than in the United States.

Social and societal disorientation is stressful, but social integration and stability is health promoting. The paradox is that all societies must and do change. At different times, in different places, and in different ways, the individuals in a society are subjected to special challenges. At these times, attention to steps that facilitate self-healing are especially valuable. A certain amount of change can produce the exhilarating "good" stress; but if emotional equilibrium is totally disrupted, *distress* and increased likelihood of illness are the result.

Some of the best evidence for the importance of social integration to health comes from extensive studies of immigrants. Interestingly, immigrants are not usually at the highest risk of disease. It is their children, the first generation to be born in the new country, who suffer the most. It seems that most immigrants are unwilling to try to adopt all of the strange customs of their new country. Rather, they move to a "Little Italy" or a "Chinatown," where cultural support is in place. Their children, however, often must face the greater stresses of leaving family traditions behind and striking out into a new culture.

COHERENCE

Viktor Frankl, the existential philosopher and therapist, developed his theories of a healing personality not in a large corporation studying executives but rather as an inmate in a Nazi concentration camp. Although most of the inmates died, the quickest to go were those who had had their sense of identity and purpose stripped away from them. Survival was more likely for those who tried living in a meaningful way, even in dire straits.

A person's sense of dignity has more than psychological and ethical importance. It is also an aspect of health. Lack of attention to this crucial factor during medical treatment seems to be what angers cancer patients the most. Much more distressing than the cancer itself is the sense of *being* a "cancer," a "tumor," a "disease." Literally hundreds of writers with cancer, representing millions of cancer victims, have pleaded over and over, "Don't talk to my spouse about me as if I'm not here"; "Don't pretend that everything is okay"; "Don't be afraid to look at me and touch me"; "Treat me as a person, not as a disease." Once a sense of dignity and meaning is gone, the will to live disappears as well.

In the last decade, the medical sociologist Aaron Antonovsky has led the fight to shift research attention from matters of disease to matters of health. He has proposed a general theory of what he calls "salutogenesis"—a theory of how people stay healthy. Central to health is a sense of coherence—a person's confidence that the world is understandable, manageable, and meaningful.

According to this approach, the world must not necessarily be controllable but controlled or ordered, in the grand scheme of things. For example, someone with a strong perception that she was carrying out God's orders may have a high sense of coherence. Dr. Antonovsky describes the case of a male survivor of the holocaust, now living in Israel. As a Jewish teenager in Nazi Europe, this individual was quite pessimistic, doubting that he would survive. Yet he had no sense of personal affront or distress—he saw all Jews in the same sinking ship and carried on with his life as best he could (including resistance efforts). After the war, it seemed natural to him that he would go to Israel and start a new life. This healthy man was hardly an optimist; rather, he had a remarkable ability to take extraordinary challenges in stride.

This understanding of meaning and dignity, more common among anthropologists and European thinkers than among ethnocentric American scientists, adds an important new twist to our comprehension of health maintenance. For self-healing personalities, life matters. In their own ways, individuals come to a view of life as ordered and clear rather than as chaotic and inexplicable. In their own way, they are intact, thriving protagonists, not isolated, alienated drifters.

SELF-HEALING

Although self-healing personalities like that shown by Bob Hope or Mohandas Gandhi are intuitively grasped, the details and implications are more complicated than they first seem. Common slogans like Be Optimistic and Don't Worry—Be Happy oversimplify and distort the true nature of the self-healing personality.

People who see everything as a lark or joke are often hiding some inner conflict that eventually may impair their homeostasis and their health. Others in the Be Happy crowd are superficial in their understanding of health and are emotionally immature; they are childlike. Their health problems arise when they first encounter significant challenge and are totally unprepared to cope with it. These are not moral judgments; they are conclusions that emerge from fifty years of personality research.

If there is a self-healing personality, then there should be all sorts of evidence for it. In the previous chapter, we analyzed the overwhelming evidence for disease-prone personalities. In the present chapter, the emphasis has been not only on avoiding disease proneness but more particularly on understanding disease resistance. Assorted studies—of health among business executives and lawyers, of the challenges of sports or unemployment, of the physiological effects of placebos, of the goals of successful psychotherapy, of disease-resistant immigrants, of recovery of patients in the hospital, and others—all point to the same conclusion. Each individual can develop a greater or lesser resistance to disease.

Importantly, it is not enough to "make up one's mind" to be healthy. Rather, a sense of control or choice in one's life, a commitment to higher goals or principles, an attitude of social integration, an environment of appropriate challenge and excitement, and a sense of creative self-fulfillment together produce the will to thrive and the positive emotions that are at the core of good health. Taken in total, the evidence for a self-healing personality is substantial.

We should not expect to see dramatic effects of self-healing in every research study. Some studies do not examine enough people, some do not continue for a long enough time, and others contain some confounding factor that obscures the true relationships. This situation is comparable, however, to the study of many other health risks, such as high blood pressure. High blood pressure is a significant risk factor for a number of diseases, but it is difficult to measure reliably, it varies over time, its effects are usually slow to accrue, and in many cases it has no obvious ill effects. Why do so many people and so many physicians worry about blood pressure but ignore emotional balance? The difference is that the traditional health care system expects to find health effects of high blood pressure, but it has not known how to think about personality and health.

The essential element of self-healing personalities is emotional equilibrium. When a degree of emotional equilibrium is maintained, the body's physiological processes can work most efficiently to keep our cells and organs functioning at their best. The challenge is to maintain this emotional equilibrium, a complex process that depends on the individual's resources and environmental demands. Fortunately, the scientific knowledge about how this can be done is now quite substantial. Specific recommendations for the individual and society are made in chapters 8 and 9.

The contemporary understanding of the self-healing personality is part of a just-beginning transformation of how society thinks about health. Recent discoveries and insights portend a dramatic reconceptualization of health and health care. The revolution is advancing rapidly in the United States, especially in California. It is not a fad; the relevant theory and research is solid and comprehensive. Rather, it is a modern scientific realization of principles of emotional balance first suggested more than two thousand years ago.

7

Inner Healing Through Nerves and Hormones

An obscure type of solid alcohol has become the most famous organic compound in the health-conscious world. Its name: cholesterol. Serum cholesterol (cholesterol in the blood) is clearly linked to heart disease. The more cholesterol in one's blood serum, the higher the risk of heart disease. The very mention of the word *cholesterol* makes some people cringe with guilt and tightness in their chests as they think of their bacon-and-eggs breakfast.

Although there is excellent scientific evidence that a high level of serum cholesterol is associated with heart disease, there is much less evidence that cholesterol is the basic *cause* of heart disease in most people. In other words, someone with a relatively low blood cholesterol level has a lower risk of heart disease, but it is not clear that most of us should be fussing so much about cholesterol itself. It is important to recognize that often it is not clear *why* any given person has a high blood cholesterol level.

The health promotion steps that a family physician recently prescribed for James, a healthy but choleric forty-year-old man with moderately high blood cholesterol, are the same ones that are appropriate for any healthy forty-year-old with *low* blood cholesterol. James was told to increase his exercise and to decrease his smoking and fat intake; unfortunately, no heed was paid to his personality. Rather than worrying about cholesterol per se, more attention should have been given to the demands on James's body and the strength of his personal resources.

For a complete understanding of the self-healing personality, a look at the physiological reverberations of psychosocial homeostasis is in order. Physiology, the study of organic processes in the body, furnishes the link, or "mechanism," between psychology and health. In particular, stressful events, the poor coping of a disease-prone personality, and the associated chronic negative emotions are closely tied to two basic physiological impairments: disturbed metabolism and weakened immune system functioning. With some simplification, current physiological work can be translated into terms a layman can understand, thereby providing a straightforward explanation of how psychological processes can affect health.

DON'T BLAME THE STEAK AND EGGS

Since eggs are cholesterol-rich, some scientists have urged us to make a drastic change in our diets—avoid eggs. However, cholesterol does not go directly from our stomachs into our blood. Besides processing the cholesterol in the food we eat, the human body makes its own cholesterol. (The body, by the way, cannot function without cholesterol.) The level of cholesterol in our blood is affected by hereditary factors, by the amount of fat (especially saturated fat) in the diet, by exercise, and by stress. It also is affected by other, as yet unknown, factors. In most people, avoiding eggs by itself will have little or no effect on serum cholesterol.

Many products on supermarket shelves are now advertising this ridiculous claim: "No cholesterol!" Believe it or not, I recently purchased a bunch of bananas that had a no cholesterol sticker attached to them. This labeling indicates a grave public misconception of the best ways to promote health.

For a whole host of reasons, it is healthy to eat lots of fruit and vegetables. Bananas do fall into this category (and I like to eat bananas), but no scientist really knows all of the exact details of why fruits and vegetables are good to eat. Certainly, a lot more than cholesterol content is involved. In fact, my judgment is that the only time it is helpful to see a no cholesterol label is when one is buying a processed food, such as graham crackers. If there is no cholesterol, then animal fat was not added to the product, which is generally a good thing. (However, this does not preclude the possibility that an unhealthy oil like coconut oil was used instead.)

Hamburgers for lunch? Red meat! A ticket to heart disease, right? Not necessarily. People's food choices and dietary changes should be evaluated in the context of their own personalities and life-styles.

I remember hearing about a family out on a trip to a regional park for a day of hiking. They got a late start, and the kids got hungry during the car ride. The kids wanted to grab a hamburger at McDonald's. But their mother was mortified at the thought of their eating "junk food" and refused to stop. The kids got hungrier, their moods soured, and they started to complain. The parents, in turn, became agitated and yelled at the children. Now, no study has ever compared the health effects of a grumpy and sullen family to the health effects of hamburgers for lunch, but my feeling is that this family would have been much better off if they had stopped for the burgers. (After all, they could have passed up the fat-laden fries and shakes in favor of salads and juices.)

How many people feel guilty when they eat a steak? The guilt is probably a greater problem than the steak. True, there is substantial evidence that high animal fat intake is unhealthy. At a restaurant near my home, I observed an obese man devour a huge fatty chunk of prime rib (the house special). He concluded the meal with a large piece of chocolate cake à la mode. If he does this often (as he evidently did), his arteries may pay the consequences. But people who occasionally enjoy eating a trimmed piece of broiled steak as part of a varied diet are giving themselves an excellent source of protein and minerals.

Not long ago, I attended a catered dinner with a group of leading cardiologists, including one eminent physician who has worked extensively on the Framingham study. (Framingham is the town in eastern Massachusetts in which a large number of residents have been followed by researchers for over thirty years. It has provided the best information we have on risk factors for heart disease.)

The dinner was served to a large group of people attending a scientific conference at a large hotel. The dinner plates appeared, covered with some kind of sauce. We guessed what was under the sauce. Most bets were on chicken, but one cardiologist guessed veal. (She figured that drug companies had made a significant monetary contribution to the conference, thus allowing the expensive veal.) Veal it was.

The big question was whether veal was an okay food. All heads turned toward the most eminent cardiologist. Like a high priest, he gave the veal his blessing and we all began to eat heartily.

I then asked him if he ever ate red meat, meaning steak and hamburger. He looked alarmed, said no, and proudly told me his low cholesterol level. But he then mentioned that his wife's cholesterol level was high, despite the fact that she shared his diet.

I asked if he thought that a no-dairy diet would be as good as a no-red-meat diet, since most dairy products are high in fat. He did not know the answer.

The American Heart Association recommends a low-fat diet to help prevent heart disease. Completely independently, the American Cancer Society recommends a low-fat diet to help prevent certain types of cancer. There is even another reason to stay away from too much fat. Evidence is starting to accumulate that diets that are high in animal fat are more likely to lead to obesity than are high-carbohydrate diets of equivalent calories. It may be the case that fat is metabolized differently or that fat tells the body to slow down its metabolism. Too much fat is unhealthy, whether in our food or on our bodies.

I believe that the National Heart, Lung, and Blood Institute, a U.S. federal agency, made a big mistake. In 1986 it instituted the National Cholesterol Program, which has had the effect of having people check to see if there is cholesterol in their bananas. What the institute should have done was institute a National *Fat* Program. Most people would be better off if they reduced their fat intake. Most people also would be better off if they simultaneously increased their daily exercise and shed excess pounds. Only a relatively few people would be helped by cholesterol screening and the ingestion of cholesterol-lowering prescription drugs. Better advice is: forget about cholesterol, think about fat.

But even this advice is somewhat misleading, because there are many people who do not have to worry about fat. They have a fast metabolism (and are not overweight), eat a variety of foods, get regular exercise, and lead active, fulfilled lives. Add in new worries about fat, and these people may wind up in worse health.

(Note: There is a small percentage of the population that suffers from hereditary conditions that produce high levels of blood cholesterol—"familial hypercholesterolemia," for example. These people usually have a parent or other close relative who had a heart attack at a young age—in their thirties or forties. Such people need to be under a cardiologist's care. But again, this is a small percentage of the population.)

This book is not about diet. So why am I saying so much about cholesterol? For two important but different reasons. First of all, it has been known for more than a generation that emotional stress can sometimes increase the cholesterol level in the blood. The more recent research is trying to work out the finer details of fat metabolism, but it is very complicated. Suffice it to say that a disease-prone personality is more likely to have metabolic problems. In some cases, high blood cholesterol and associated atherosclerotic problems are promoted by emotional struggle. In other cases, the cholesterol level is not too high but rather drops too low, a finding that is associated with the development of cancer. In other words, making people worried about cholesterol and paranoid about their food is no way to improve health; there are various causes of impaired metabolic processes. On the other hand, a person with a self-healing personality and good general health habits is likely to do just fine.

But isn't maintaining a low-cholesterol diet far more important than emotional health? Not at all! Research suggests that the associations between chronic negative emotions and health are just as large as the associations between particular aspects of diet and health. People have been misled by the confusion between cholesterol in the diet and cholesterol in the blood.

The second reason for my attention to cholesterol is to warn against overly simple solutions to complex problems. The case of cholesterol illustrates the complexity of the physiological bases of good health. Just as the influences of diet on physiological processes relevant to heart disease and cancer are not simple, the physiological elements of emotional balance also are not simple. Doctors who advise their patients to "be optimistic" are grossly oversimplifying the scientific evidence.

In short, just as diet affects the body's metabolism, so, too, is it affected by emotional balance. There are many ways in which the activities of our nerves and our hormones, influenced by stress, affect the body's processes of energy storage, release, and utilization.

SYMPATHETIC AROUSAL

The sympathetic nervous system is that part of the nervous system most involved in negative reactions to stress. It is easy to learn to see what happens to this system when a disease-prone person is challenged.

Consider the case of Ray, a classic choleric man of sixty. I studied his style on videotape. Whenever Ray felt he was getting a raw deal, his eyebrows were drawn down and inward toward his nose. His pupils dilated. His mouth and lips became tense and firm, often with teeth clenched. His voice changed as his mouth dried out and his vocal cords tensed up. I could sense his increased heart rate and faster breathing—he was ready to fight. Ray's sympathetic nervous system was firing away.

Louise was a fifty-year-old phlegmatic who repressed her feelings. When her sympathetic nervous system was activated, her outward reactions were more restrained. Her face showed a forced smile and her skin changed color. Her body tensed, but in a closed position. She refused to look others in the eye. An observer could not detect it, but her blood pressure rose, her skin conductance rose, and she felt palpitations (flutterings) in her heart.

Mary was sanguine and enthusiastic, while Joan was melancholic. Both were schoolteachers. Initially they reacted similarly when their sympathetic systems were activated. Their jaws dropped, their eyes widened, their stomachs churned, and they began to fidget. But as tears came to their eyes, their reaction patterns diverged. Joan would become more and more distressed and might tremble all day. Mary, on the other hand, would take a deep breath, stretch her muscles, and begin to regain her equilibrium.

Prolonged sympathetic activation is unhealthy, for a variety of reasons. Although the precise links to disease have not yet been completely identified, there are several likely paths.

First, sympathetic arousal usually raises blood pressure, and high blood pressure is a significant risk factor for heart disease and stroke. (It was the Framingham study that first offered substantial evidence that high blood pressure—hypertension—is a significant risk factor for cardiovascular disease.) Why does hypertension sometimes lead to cardiovascular disease? No one knows for sure, but the scientific reasoning currently goes as follows.

It is a fact that atherosclerosis (plaque buildup in the blood vessels) occurs in arteries but usually not in veins. (The only time buildup is likely in veins is when they are used as arteries in coronary bypass operations.) Arteries carry blood away from the heart and are under high pressure. By the time the blood reaches the veins, the pressure is much lower. This and other evidence suggests that it is the high pressure itself that encourages the buildup of fatty plaques on the artery walls. The high pressure, even if temporary, may damage the artery walls directly, facilitate the deposit of fats in the artery wall, or both. Sometimes the high pressure causes a different kind of problem—a blood vessel in the brain ruptures, producing a stroke (cerebral hemorrhage).

These events are amplified by disruptions in the normal internal regulatory processes, in an ongoing cycle. For example, activation of the sympathetic nervous system also stimulates the adrenal gland, a hormone center located on the kidney. The medulla (middle) of the adrenal gland then releases catecholamines (such as adrenaline), hormones that travel through the body, maintaining the sympathetic arousal and changing the body's usual biochemical reactions. This shot of adrenaline is what one feels when suddenly frightened or, in a literal sense, when given a novocaine anesthetic injection by a dentist (often the injection also contains adrenaline). When challenged, choleric Type As have especially intense changes in their systolic blood pressure and their catecholamine (norepinephrine) levels.

Occasionally the electrical rhythms of the heartbeat are thereby disrupted, resulting in ventricular fibrillation (uncontrolled fluttering) and sudden death. This type of sudden death may occur even in a young person with no artery disease, although plaque deposits make it more likely.

THE CORTISOL PROCESS

To really view the complete picture, one other very important physiological system must be added. It is usually termed the pituitary-adreno-cortical axis, or simply the cortisol process. Cortisol is a steroid, the body's internal form of the hydrocortisone cream that one might apply to a skin rash. Cortisol and its sister chemicals are hormones (from the Greek *hormon*, "to set in motion")—so called because they travel throughout the body activating all sorts of physiological processes.

What causes cortisol to be released? When the body is challenged (internally or externally), information about the challenge is sent to the brain. The brain's response depends on one's personality and coping mechanisms. If the challenge is seen as a threat to internal balance, this information is communicated through the hypothalamus area of the brain to the pituitary. The pituitary is the body's master gland, located in the base of the brain.

The pituitary in turn sends out hormones that stimulate the adrenal cortex, part of the gland on the kidney. Then the adrenal cortex secretes the cortisol. The cortisol tries to help the body reestablish an internal homeostasis. All sorts of psychological stresses, including guilt, bereavement, and repressed anxiety, have been shown to raise cortisol levels. The results of this process are monitored continually by the brain, which may direct the release of more or less cortisol.

Although the details are complicated, the concepts are simple: The body does not function in a linear or mechanical manner. It is not the case that psychological stress "breaks" the body like physical stress may break one's arm or leg. Rather, the body is a live system, constantly struggling to maintain its equilibrium. When these concepts are understood, it becomes easier to think in terms of a self-healing personality.

Is cortisol good or bad? Yes—cortisol is both good and bad. Cortisol fights inflammations. Steroid drugs like cortisone are among the most powerful tools in the physician's pharmacopoeia. Cortisol also maintains a necessary biochemical responsiveness of blood vessels and helps regulate the balance of water in the body. What happens if you encounter stress or illness with low levels of cortisol and its sister hormones? The result is hypotension, shock, and death.

On the bad side, cortisol can interfere with fat (fatty acid) mobilization, thus accelerating the atherosclerotic process. It also can significantly depress the immune system. Remember, too, that very high levels of cortisol go hand in hand with major psychological depression. In severe emotional distress, it appears that the feedback mechanism has broken down and the supply of cortisol cannot be turned off. All sorts of problems can result.

So cortisol in the right amount and at the right time is healthy; but when a major emotional imbalance throws the cortisol system out of whack, the effects of this and related hormones can be quite dangerous.

Let us return to the matter of stress and cholesterol. How is stress involved with cholesterol levels and heart disease? Both the sympathetic nervous system and the cortisol system are involved. Disease-prone individuals are more likely to show increased nervous system and hormonal system response when subjected to challenge. In turn, catecholamines, such as adrenaline, affect the activity of the heart and arteries; the excess activity may change or injure the lining of the arteries, permitting blockages to form. The released hormones simultaneously affect the metabolism of fats and cholesterol, and it is these fats that are deposited in the arteries to form atherosclerotic plaque (hardened arteries).

The exact details of the atherosclerotic process—the topics of lipid metabolism, high- and low-density lipoproteins, and so on—are receiving intensive study and should be well documented during the next decade. Low-density lipoprotein (LDL) cholesterol is the "bad" cholesterol that promotes formation of plaque in the arteries. High-density lipoprotein (HDL) is the "good" cholesterol that helps remove fatty deposits. How can we lower the bad stuff and increase the good stuff? The most intense research efforts are now being directed at doing so through expensive and sometimes-dangerous drugs. However, I predict that emotional and behavioral modifications eventually will be shown to be safe and effective in accomplishing the same thing for many people.

Much less well understood is the relationship of metabolic processes to cancer development. It is well established that serum cholesterol is inversely associated with the development of cancer; and it is suspected that cancer development is sometimes promoted by a metabolic disturbance involving the body's utilization of fatty acids in the blood. But the causal links have not yet been isolated. Most important, however, it is well established that cortisol directly affects the immune system processes, those processes that defend us against cancer.

IMMUNITY FROM PERSECUTION

When we face divorce or the death of a loved one, we feel the physical shock to our bodies. We may become weak or sickly, suffer heartache and pain. This has been recognized for thousands of years. But often these deeply felt shocks are dismissed as "emotional distress." Until now, we did not know how to link them to physical illness.

In addition to the cortisol and nervous systems, the primary physiological system of the human body relevant to health is the immune system. New research shows that these systems are all interrelated and often interdependent. As one system is thrown out of equilibrium, others may be affected. It was a major recent breakthrough to discover that the immune system, which protects us from invading bacteria and viruses, does not work independently but rather is closely tied to our thoughts (psychology) and the reactions of our nerves and brain (neurology).

This new field of study is thus termed psychoneuroimmunology. The term is quite a mouthful, but this is the field in which future Nobel Prizes are now being earned. Unfortunately, sometimes the word *psychoneuroimmunology* is waved around like a magic wand. Knowing that our minds affect our immunities does not by itself insure that we will develop a self-healing personality.

I have seen dentists trying psychoneuroimmunology to cure toothaches and chiropractors using it to try to cure back pain. Despite the high potential of this approach, unless its limits are clearly understood and its effectiveness demonstrated for a given application, it easily could become another Krebiozen or Laetrile fad.

What happens when the body encounters cells that should not be there, such as invading bacteria or cancer? The body's immune system tries to fight off the infection or cancer with exotic-sounding cells called T cells, B cells, and natural killer (NK) cells. For example, it is T cells that are weakened by the AIDS virus, thus allowing rare cancers and unusual infections to grow. On the other hand, when immune cells are too responsive, they may attack harmless cells, thereby exacerbating allergies, asthma, and arthritis.

Despite the horror of the AIDS virus, there is a much more common threat to our immune cells: stress. Stress reactions result in the release of high levels of hormones that interfere with the actions of immune system cells. The hormone cortisol, for instance, suppresses the immune system.

It took a long time for the direct links between stress and immunity to be discovered. There were a number of reasons for this, but I think the most important reason was that some scientists were studying only cells but not people, while other scientists were investigating stressed people but not their immune cells. Finally, in 1977 an important study of the physiological consequences of bereavement compared the immune system responses of healthy people who had unexpectedly lost their spouses to the responses of a control group of people of the same age. The researchers found that the responsiveness of the immune system fell dramatically about two months after the bereavement. More recent investigations have found that bereavement affects other immune functions—for example, recently bereaved women have significantly lower NK cell activity than comparable women whose husbands are healthy.

However, such research also finds hints that becoming depressed after bereavement (not merely losing a spouse) is related to the impaired immune activity. This finding is consistent with the large body of evidence that suggests a relationship between general depression (or repressed feelings) and impaired immune system functioning. In other words, the relationship between life challenges and immune system–related disease is more likely to emerge in people with a melancholic or phlegmatic, disease-prone personality. This type of finding provides the physiological basis for explaining the difference between the widowed breast cancer victim who succumbs and the one who recovers.

This all makes physiological sense because of the discovery of paths that link the brain and the immune system. The brain communicates to the immune cells, and the immune cells in turn send messages back to the brain (through peptide hormones). The nervous system has been traced to the centers where lymphocytes are made. Further, the central nervous system and the immune system share cell-surface receptors for various hormones. Immunity has now taken its place next to the other physiological systems that form vast feedback loops, with the brain at the center of activity.

What does this mean in practice? Under stress, the release of catecholamines (such as adrenaline) may interfere with the actions of lymphocytes (white blood cells); physiological receptors for stress hormones have been found on lymphocytes. The impaired immune function may then result in the increased likelihood of illness, such as colds and flu. The actual process is undoubtedly somewhat more complicated, since stress and viruses are not perfectly related to colds and flu. But all of the important links already have been shown to exist.

No one is immune from persecution. We constantly face internal and external threats to our equilibrium, whether we recognize them or not. But some people are generally more resistant to ("immune from") disease; their internal coping system can quickly reestablish harmony. The immune system is a very complex one, however, and any doctor who regularly claims simple cures by means of psychological intervention is overstating the evidence.

Detailed knowledge of the immune system is not necessary for understanding the essentials of a self-healing personality. In any case, the exact physiological mechanisms have not yet been fully discovered. Some psychologists and psychiatrists hail the neuroimmunologists as holding the keys to a long and healthy life. What do the neuroimmunologists themselves say? Many think that the important answers in psychoneuroimmunology are likely to come from psychology.

MONKEYS, BABOONS, AND RABBITS

As discussed earlier in this book, it is very stressful for an aggressive, domineering businessperson to move away to a new community, with the stress of a new job and the need to reestablish control. It turns out that the same is true for monkeys. In captive monkeys, however, physiological changes can be more easily assessed; you do not need to make an appointment.

In one experiment, researchers studied thirty adult male monkeys for almost two years. Half of the monkeys lived in stable, five-animal groups. The other monkeys also lived in small groups, but the researchers kept changing the composition of the groups. So these monkeys had to keep repeating their struggle for dominance. They did indeed struggle and fight and reestablish dominance each time the group changed.

During this time, the monkeys' behavior, physiology, and social status were closely observed. At the end of the two years it was found that it was the dominant (high-status), aggressive monkeys of the unstable, shifting social groups that were much more likely to have atherosclerosis.

In a follow-up study, all of the monkeys were kept on a low-fat, low-cholesterol diet. But some were again put into stressful, unstable groups. It was found that although the overall rate of atherosclerosis was lower for these diet-controlled monkeys, the stressed, high-status monkeys were still likely to develop clogged arteries. The repeated struggle was unhealthy.

What characterized the responses of those monkeys most likely to develop atherosclerosis? There is no generally accepted measure of monkey personality. (Don't laugh—the idea has been seriously considered.) However, changes in a monkey's heart rate in response to challenge can easily be monitored, and monkeys (like people) differ markedly on this variable. It turns out that those aggressive, "high heart rate reactor" monkeys were the most likely to develop severe atherosclerosis. We cannot know for sure, but it is a good guess that they had choleric personalities.

Let us turn now to baboons. Olive baboons are highly social primates and live in large groups. As in humans, male baboons form dominance hierarchies, and they may compete aggressively. Interesting work by Dr. Robert Sapolsky in a protected reserve in Kenya shows important individual differences among baboons. In these stable groups, the higher-ranking males, who exerted control over the group's activities, were less affected physiologically by stress than were the low-ranking male baboons.

It may not be a topic for polite conversation, but ill people often judge their degree of illness by their sexual responsiveness. A good sign of recovery from a serious illness is the return of sexual desires, and an ongoing problem for many chronically ill people is the diminution of sexual desires. These changes are due to a variety of physiological factors, but one of the most important in men is the level of the hormone testosterone, which stimulates and maintains male sex characteristics, sperm production, and general bodily growth and development. It would be an oversimplification to say that more is better, but deficiencies in testosterone due to castration or illness lead to marked changes in strength and potency.

Getting back to Dr. Sapolsky's baboons, it is interesting to observe the effects of stress on baboon testosterone. These baboons, living freely in East Africa, were watched closely for several months and then captured for examination (using anesthesia). During the first hour following the stress of being captured for examination, the high- and low-ranking males differed dramatically in physiological responses. The testosterone concentrations of the high-status males rose, while that of the low-ranking males fell. Further investigation suggested that the difference was due to the effects of—guess what—the sympathetic nervous system. The psychological aspects of being a dominant male baboon in a stable social setting seemed to directly affect the body's reaction to stress.

Baboon cholesterol? In a related study, the blood concentrations of HDL cholesterol—the so-called good cholesterol—of the low-status male baboons was found to be much lower than that of dominant baboons, possibly due to stress-induced elevations in cortisol levels. These baboon observations thus support the findings collected on monkeys, but they add further confirmation of the stress-related physiological mechanisms.

Even New Zealand rabbits cannot escape the advance of medical science. In a recent study, various combinations of rabbits were induced to develop (or not develop) atherosclerosis and then were subjected (or not subjected) to stress. The interesting result was that the combination of stress and atherosclerosis produced far greater alterations in fat (lipid) metabolism than did either stress or atherosclerosis alone.

This finding is consistent with evidence that suggests that it is not only one's personality that influences reactions to challenge but also the current physical state of the body. Stress-induced imbalance will likely have greater effects on physiological processes that already have begun to go awry. This is part of the reason why not everyone with a disease-prone personality becomes ill. It also helps explain why psychosocial factors often have a greater effect on recovery from illness than they do on the development of illness.

Health buffs know that we can get a lot more detailed than a simple consideration of cholesterol levels. One key index involves the ratio of LDLs to HDLs. Even here, there is evidence for direct effects of changing social status and stress, and the research was done on humans. One prospective study examined more than four hundred blue-collar workers in terms of job instability and perceived job pressures. As expected, those men suffering from chronic occupational instability and stress had significantly worse lipoprotein ratios. These results held constant even after taking into account differences in weight, age, smoking habits, and alcohol use.

THE GOOD PHYSIOLOGICAL RESPONSES

Athletes who have good cardiovascular fitness not only have greater speed and endurance, they also have the ability to recover quickly. For example, they have an easier time catching their breath. In physiological terms, they are better able to reestablish internal homeostasis. The final physiological proof has not yet been gathered, but it is a good bet that a self-healing personality has the ability to return quickly to an emotional homeostasis. We might say that those with healing personalities can more easily "capture their equilibrium."

Following this line of thought, we should expect *protective* physiological activity in self-healing individuals, not just a lessened tendency toward physiological disruption. For example, true Type B individuals, who presumably do not suffer the harmful physiological effects of stress, should have an emotionally fit nervous system. In fact, some recent research does indeed find this to be the case. Type B individuals seem to have more active "heart-calming" nervous systems. That is, it is not only the case that Type As overreact to stress, it is also that Type Bs have especially active calming or restorative systems.

Heroin addicts usually develop an interesting set of symptoms. Sex drive plummets. Heart rate slows. Digestion and appetite are disturbed. Pain temporarily disappears. And, of course, mood swings wildly from euphoria to desperation. All of these effects and others are caused by the actions of the heroin on opiate receptors in the brain and nervous system. Not surprisingly, since these effects sometimes can occur without any heroin, the body has been found to have its own internal opiate system of *endo*genous *morphine*s, called endorphins. It is probable that healing personalities have a stable system of endorphin release that corrects bodily challenges and then returns to homeostasis.

I was always intrigued by the case of Kay, who twice developed both gallstones and high cholesterol levels after periods of intense stress. My puzzlement disappeared when I read a series of studies of endorphins in mice. There is good evidence that both gallstone formation and high blood cholesterol are encouraged by disturbances in the central endorphin system. In fact, when an endorphin blocker ("opiate antagonist") called naltrexone is administered to mice, the detrimental effects of stress are reversed.

In general, however, the special physiological strengths of the self-healing personality have not been studied much. Why bother to study healthy people when we have so many ill people to worry about? This short-sighted philosophy is a natural result of our inadequate conceptions of health. Although we have seen that the self-healing personality is not merely the absence of a disease-prone personality, the physiological aspects of this distinction have not yet been fully documented. This may change with the increasing scientific attention to the brain's chemicals and wave patterns.

THE BRAIN, THE UNCONSCIOUS, AND HEALTH

Most people know that Sigmund Freud brought the idea of an unconscious into scientific and popular thinking at the beginning of the twentieth century. (His book *The Interpretation of Dreams* was published, by his own design, in the year 1900.) As the beginning of the twenty-first century approaches, have we advanced beyond Freud's conceptions? Indeed we have, although sometimes it is hard to tell.

As he treated his patients, Freud began to notice that they often did not seem to understand the emotions that were troubling them. They might have experienced an emotional trauma, such as being molested as a young child, but could not remember it. In other words, they did not have access to what was in their own minds. However, Dr. Freud found evidence of these emotional conflicts through his patients' dreams, through hypnosis, through slips of the tongue, and eventually through a well-developed system of psychoanalysis. When the emotional conflict was resolved, the patient often felt better, both physically and mentally.

Freud explained these feelings as existing in the unconscious, a place where threatening thoughts were hidden, in the deep recesses of the mind. They were pushed there by the superego, a conscience that protects us from the base, animal urges contained in the id. Freud was correct in proposing that children are socialized by society to control their biological urges, and that an inner tension can result. There is little doubt that sometimes we do have hidden emotional conflicts that we cannot easily access through our conscious thought processes. But is Freud's model the best one? Probably not.

The Freudian model leads us to think in terms of repressed memories struggling to get out, changed memories distorted by intellectualization processes, and so on. Modern psychobiology suggests a more accurate model.

Multiple Brains

Think of the brain as a vast system of smaller brains. These smaller brains communicate with one another to some extent, but they also specialize in and concentrate on their own particular tasks. The brain is actually a multiple brain.

What kind of evidence is there for this multiple-brain model? First, there are various different physical structures in the brain. For example, there is the left hemisphere of the brain, which generally controls language and analytic thought; and there is the right hemisphere, which is more involved with spatial issues, images, and artistic abilities. Each hemisphere does not know what the other hemisphere is "thinking" unless the information is sent across the nerve bridge known as the corpus callosum. (This transfer is usually automatic. We know that the two hemispheres can think independently, however, through studies of patients whose corpus callosum has been severed during a surgical procedure.)

Second, there is evolutionary evidence for the idea of multiple brains. Higher and lower animals contain the primitive central core of the brain, containing basic structures like the cerebellum, which controls muscle coordination, and the hypothalamus, which controls metabolism. The primitive brain lets a fish swim or a person walk. More highly evolved animals—mammals—have brains that also contain the limbic system. The limbic system lets the animal override basic instincts, learn from experience, and be more adaptable. The most highly evolved animals have a cerebrum in their brains; this allows more complex sensation and thought.

We do not have to think to keep our heart beating and our lungs breathing; primitive parts of our brains control these functions automatically. In fact, it is difficult to try to consciously speed up or slow down our heart rate. The different parts of the brain communicate with one another but evolved separately. Unlike an IBM computer, there is no master blueprint or grand design for the brain. Many things can go on in the vast expanse of our brains without any awareness on our part.

A third kind of evidence for the idea of multiple brains appears when someone develops a brain disease. If a stroke or a tumor destroys part of the brain, there is not a general decrement in performance; rather, there are often peculiar, distinct impairments. For example, some stroke patients can speak but cannot understand others; other patients can understand others but cannot speak. Some patients become emotional, but others lose all emotion, depending on the part of the brain that is damaged. Some patients become obsessive. Some lose the ability to understand nouns (but not verbs). Others become disoriented. There is tremendous differentiation in the brain.

This idea of multiple brains should not be taken too far. The parts of the brain are interconnected. In fact, sometimes one part of the brain can take over a function for another part of the brain. But it is also true that each part of the brain evolved and grew to function somewhat independently. There can be a breakdown in the homeostasis of one part of the body without there being direct effects on other parts of the body.

The idea of multiple brains is so important to the self-healing personality because it leads to the understanding that we can have internal imbalances of which we are unaware. Freud called them unconscious conflicts. I prefer the imagery of unresolved imbalances.

In a recent study, a thirty-three-year-old Vietnam veteran described how he saw his buddy's head blown off by the machine-gun fire of a female enemy soldier. Shocked and incensed at the sudden killing of his friend, the soldier then chased the enemy down, shot her in the leg, ripped off her clothes, and raped her. Hearing the approach of American helicopters, he pulled out his knife and slit the woman's throat.

This episode was reported to psychologist James Pennebaker, who was studying the relationship between emotional inhibition and disease. Dr. Pennebaker has found that many people carry around deep, dark secrets that they have mostly "forgotten." When prompted, however, many people are more than willing to dredge up the terrors, little by little. The general finding of these studies is that the more the emotional traumas are talked about or written about, the less distress the people feel and the healthier they seem. The disclosure is not immediately uplifting—on the contrary, it is usually somewhat depressing. But the long-term effect is for better physical and mental health. Together this suggests that an emotional balance is slowly being restored. Most interesting for the present discussion, links are found to both nervous system activity levels and to immune system responsiveness. In simple terms, people who disclose troubling experiences that they have previously held back soon begin to show decreased sympathetic activity (decreased fight-or-flight activation) and increased immune system activity. And in general, recent research suggests that depressed people and psychiatrically disturbed people have disrupted immune systems. These results thus provide an interesting window on the direct relationships between hidden conflicts, physiological responses, and health.

Undoubtedly the whole picture is somewhat more complicated than has just been described. As the body faces challenges, some internal systems first increase and later decrease in activity, while others do the reverse. Further, since several systems are reacting simultaneously, simple isolated effects often are not found. But the probable links to health are clear enough. In fact, the recent conclusion of a number of the world's leading experts on emotions, with each scientist using an independent approach, is that internal emotional conflicts will damage one's physical health.

PHYSIOLOGICAL LINKS
TO OUR MAJOR HEALTH THREATS

What are the direct links to health and disease? It may be helpful at this point to consider the major threats to the health of the population, with regard to relevance of the disease-prone and self-healing personalities in causing pertinent physiological changes.

When asked about diseases they fear, some people report concern about getting disabling diseases like Lou Gehrig's disease (amyotrophic lateral sclerosis). Such paralyzing conditions are quite striking and salient, and we remember them when we hear about them. But in fact, such conditions are rare. Residents of the industrialized world are far more likely to suffer a fatal heart attack or be killed in a car crash. In other words, people worry about the wrong threats to their health.

Cardiovascular disease is by far the greatest killer. Cardiovascular (literally, "heart vessel") diseases are mainly heart attacks and strokes. As discussed earlier, the narrowing of the arteries that supply the heart and brain is facilitated by the actions of the sympathetic nervous system and the cortisol system. In particular, the stress hormones (especially catecholamines and cortisol) have repeatedly been shown to be relevant to cardiovascular disease processes. Even minor reductions in cardiovascular disease due to increased knowledge of the self-healing personality (and proper corrective measures) will produce tremendous improvements in health status and great monetary savings, since cardiovascular disease is such a tremendous threat.

Until the advent of AIDS, *cancer* was cited repeatedly as people's greatest fear. It is not just one of the most-feared diseases, it is also one of the greatest fears, period. In statistical terms, people have good reason to fear cancer. Cancer is the cause of about one-fifth of all deaths in Western societies. We use the term *cancer* in the singular, but cancer is actually a number of different diseases, all involving the uncontrolled growth of cells. The exact causes of cancer are still unknown, although genetic defects, viruses, and cell damage from external sources (such as radiation) are known to play a role in many cancers.

As we have seen, there is good evidence that the body's immune system protects it from some developing cancers. The cortisol system and perhaps also the sympathetic nervous system can suppress the immune system. There is more. In addition to the failure of an impaired immune system in destroying incipient cancers, there is some evidence, gathered by psychoimmunologists Janice Kiecolt-Glaser and Ronald Glaser, that psychological distress suppresses the body's normal repair of damaged DNA in cells. If the DNA is not repaired, cancer seems to be a possible result.

Behavior also plays an important role here. Cigarettes and other pollutants and poisons are responsible for a large number of cancer cases. In a clean environment without tobacco smoke, lung cancer (the single greatest cause of cancer death) would be rare. Similarly, toxic chemicals and radiation can cause many other cancers, especially in genetically vulnerable people. To a large extent, changes in behavior that help people avoid carcinogens can be effective in helping people avoid cancer. These effects are separate from and in addition to the physiological effects of the healing personality on increasing one's resistance to cancer. But healthy behaviors generally go hand in hand with emotionally stable personalities.

When Rock Hudson, the glamorous movie star, died of AIDS (acquired immunodeficiency syndrome), the Western world suddenly woke up to the danger posed by this deadly disease. For some people, AIDS poses virtually no risk. Monogamous couples (or sexually abstinent people) who do not receive blood transfusions or share dirty needles are not at risk. On the other hand, many of their neighbors are at high risk. AIDS is spread primarily through behavior, and there is some suggestion that its course can be affected by psychological influences. Something must account for the fact that the incubation period for AIDS is so variable from person to person; perhaps internal emotional imbalance plays a role.

AIDS is an interesting example for the present discussion, for it illustrates both the power and the limits of the self-healing personality. Can a healing personality fight AIDS? At the simplest level, to the extent that people are psychologically fulfilled and well adapted, they are more likely to behave in ways that will help them prevent becoming infected or that will maintain their general health. Although there are some ongoing studies of the direct influence of psychological state on the progression of AIDS in infected people, there is ample evidence indicating that this disease is heavily biologically determined. That is, most people are very likely to become infected if their blood is exposed to sufficient quantities of the virus, and once infected, they are very likely to develop AIDS. Once full-blown AIDS develops, they are very likely to die within a few years. However, at least some patients manage to outlive the norms. Just as someone with an exceptionally strong, efficient heart is more likely to resist threats to the heart, so, too, is it reasonable to expect that a well-balanced immune system will be better able to resist the AIDS virus, at least for a while. The jury, however, is still out on this point.

Future research on physiological aspects of the self-healing personality is likely to focus increasingly on the liver, a large chemical factory that produces many substances essential for life. The liver controls the amount of sugar and fat in the blood, and it removes harmful materials like alcohol from the blood. It also controls the amount of cholesterol in our blood. When a liver fails, very little can be done to save the patient. As a key organ in internal balance, the liver is heavily involved when there is emotional disruption.

Hepatitis, or inflammation of the liver, is a common disease, usually caused by a virus. Chronic hepatitis can lead to cirrhosis, a progressive destruction of the liver. However, most cirrhosis of the liver is due to excessive consumption of alcohol. The interactions among alcohol, stress hormones, and liver function have not yet been studied extensively, but I do not know any eighty-year-old drunks. (The amiable old drunk stereotyped in films may *look* eighty but is probably more like forty.)

Anyone who teaches or works around college students, graduate students, or medical students knows that colds, flus, and lung infections peak around exam times. Influenza is a viral infection of the upper respiratory tract. Pneumonia is an inflammation of the lungs. Both are serious and are major health threats. A number of studies of students have shown that several aspects of the immune system are suppressed at these stressful exam times. Then again, sometimes the virus is just too strong for anyone's immune system to resist.

Diabetes, involving deficiencies in the hormone insulin, is another major cause of illness. (The pancreas works with the liver to control blood sugar.) Lack of insulin can result in too much sugar in the blood.

If too much insulin is taken, then low blood sugar can result. Diabetes is a major cause of disability and death. Because diabetes is an endocrine disorder, it is sometimes closely related to stress responses. Some cases of diabetes can be cured solely by stress management and exercise.

Although the causes of diabetes are not fully understood, it can be triggered by infections, by excessive stress, by certain drugs, or by other hormonal changes, such as those that occur during pregnancy. There is also some evidence that immune system deficiencies are relevant to diabetes. Furthermore, once diabetes develops, psychological changes are not uncommon, since blood sugar is related to faintness, irritability, trembling, drowsiness, anxiety, and similar states. Stress does not *cause* diabetes, but there is increasing evidence that emotional homeostasis often plays a key part in blood glucose homeostasis. Here the positive effects of "good stress" should not be forgotten— fascination and curiosity can moderate the effects of blood sugar fluctuations, as any grumpy, exhausted traveler who finally reaches a wonderful vacation destination can tell you.

Chronic conditions, such as arthritis, migraines, ulcers, asthma, and headache, afflict millions of people. As we have seen, all are associated with the disease-prone personality. In all of these conditions, disruptions in the immune system, the sympathetic nervous system, or both have been implicated as a causal factor. For example, many asthmatics suffer from other immune-related disorders, such as food allergies, eczema, or allergic rhinitis. Thus, on the basis of the physiological evidence, it should not be surprising that all of these conditions can be helped through the development of a self-healing personality.

In short, major threats to health are not primarily from invading bacteria or natural bodily deteriorations which internists and surgeons are well trained to treat. Medical care (especially antibiotic drugs) and preventive public health measures (primarily sewage control and immunization) already have controlled most of those threats. Rather, the new challenges to health come from internal bodily processes gone awry; they also come from external physical traumas.

Behavior-related Influences

Although most of them do not know it, for young or middle-aged adults living in the suburbs, the greatest threat to health comes from *automobile accidents*. In fact, when loss of years of life is taken into account, accidental death and injury are the greatest threats to the health of the American population.

Why talk about accidents in a book about the healing personality? When a tractor trailer rig is bearing down on your compact sedan, it really does not matter whether you have meditated or eaten enough vegetables, whether you are choleric or melancholic—right? Right, but our view of health should not be too limited. First, emotionally distressed or imbalanced people are more likely to have accidents. Second, personality affects preventive behaviors, such as using seat belts. Many injuries and premature deaths could be eliminated through a better understanding of people and their place in their environments.

Other accidents are also a major threat to health. Not plane crashes, but simple things, like falls, cuts, and burns. And although fires are a significant factor in burns, they are by no means the only factor. For example, scald burns caused by hot tap water result in thousands of hospitalizations. Ironically, many so-called accidents are not really accidents at all.

Much progress already has been made in this area, often at low cost. Children are protected by safe cribs, inspected toys, childproof bottle caps, car seats, and so on. On the other hand, the elderly have not been protected much from slippery bathrooms, dangerous stairways, hazardous street crossings, poorly designed cooking and heating systems, and so on. For most of the population, far more could be done to design and match the environment to fit with the ways people behave.

Suicide is a major cause of death in Western society and is an especially great factor in total years of life lost. In discussing personality and health, a common first impulse is to try to exclude suicide. Suicide is not a disease. On further thought, however, many relevant issues arise. Many suicide victims suffered somatic symptoms, such as chronic pain, which are known to be intensified by emotional state. Many suicide victims suffered from major depression. And many suicide victims gave up on life because they felt they could not adapt to the world. All of these issues are relevant to the healing personality.

The final behavior-related threat is *homicide*. For black males in the United States, homicide is a leading killer. Violence is also an important cause of death and disability for young white males. As with accidents and suicide, homicide, of course, has much more to do with human behavior than with the immune system or catecholamines. But here again, reductions in emotional imbalances that go hand in hand with smoother interpersonal relations will have a salutary effect on the homicide rate.

In short, all of the main threats to health are known to be linked, one way or another, to personality. Some traditional medical analysts are willing to concede that emotional imbalance is relevant to physical health, but they believe it is a minor factor. As we approach the problems of health care in the twenty-first century, I cannot think of a greater factor.

The physiological evidence for the self-healing personality is here, even though few clinicians are looking for it. It is ironic that while some poorly informed physicians and psychologists still are debating whether stress really affects health, physiologists are accepting stress-induced physiological disturbance as a given.

Once the relevance of distress to disease is accepted, the battle is only half won. Some researchers and many individuals overlook the forest for the trees. The lesson to be learned is that it is not necessary to worry obsessively about whether one has eaten enough carrots and bran today. Such worries lead to diets that people cannot remember or follow, and they divert attention from the broader view of a healthy life-style.

The solution does not involve worrying about emotional imbalance as we now worry improperly about cholesterol in bananas. Rather, just as the significance of a microbe invasion depends on the body's physiological responsiveness, so, too, must the individual's resources be examined in terms of the situational demands placed on those resources. Ways of creating a better match between resources and demands is the subject of the next chapter.

8

Achieving Homeostasis: Developing a Self-healing Personality

The good news concerning disease-prone personalities is that they can be changed into self-healing personalities. People can and do become better able to cope with their environments and mend their disease-promoting emotional imbalances. And years of psychotherapy are not necessary. *But most people misunderstand what is beneficial.*

Benjamin Franklin, in whimsical discussions with his gout, pleads with his gout to leave him alone: "I promise faithfully never more to play at chess, but to take exercise daily and live temperately." The gout responds, "You promise fair, but after a few months of good health, you will return to your old habits." Analogously, one big mistake most disease-prone people make is that they try to change their negative feelings directly, through promises. People resolve, "I'm going to try to be less tense and uptight." Or they proclaim, "I'm going to worry less, and I'm going to lose some weight," or "I'm going to be more cheerful and optimistic," or "From now on, I won't worry so much about my work—it's only a job." As Ben Franklin knew, most such resolutions fail miserably within about six months.

Doctors and therapists also sometimes head down the wrong path. They advise patients, "Don't worry so much," "Stop those negative thoughts," "Be reasonable." If people could readily take such advice, they would not have come seeking help in the first place. The truth is that simple slogans do not work for most people in most situations. Too many people miss the boat by thinking we can simply will our way to health.

Even worse, some patients are given (or find) tranquilizers and other drugs for psychosocial difficulties. (The medical journals have large color ads for all sorts of "new and improved" mind-altering drugs.) This is like giving lung-altering drugs to people breathing smoggy air instead of cleaning up the air, or like giving weight-loss pills to a laxative-gobbling, binging-purging bulimic. Tranquilizers are sometimes very useful for short-term treatment of a major crisis, but over a period of months they become still another personal problem.

Sally was an alcoholic middle-aged woman and respected member of her community, who repeatedly and unsuccessfully vowed to her family to go on the wagon. She died of a stroke exacerbated by liver disease. Such cases are familiar to almost everyone. Willpower alone occasionally is effective in overcoming unhealthy behaviors, but relapse is by far the more common outcome. The same is true for personality imbalances. A healing personality can be developed, but *not* through force of will alone.

The second key mistake most people make is that they fail to evaluate which changes are best for them as individuals. The same advice to buy a Walkman and go jogging would not be suitable for both an anxious, competitive twenty-five-year-old businessman with migraines and a depressed, isolated sixty-year-old woman with breast cancer. Solutions must be tailored for the needs of the individual. This is obvious when stated but too often ignored in practice.

Two case histories from my studies are especially relevant here. The first case concerns a competitive and choleric fifty-year-old executive, Sam, who worked all the time and seemed to become progressively more worn out, pale, and sickly looking. Rather than recognizing his chronic hostility as the problem, Sam's wife (with support from his doctor) nagged him until he agreed to take a month-long vacation in Hawaii. The forced change in routine was so stressful that it was the final straw—Sam promptly had a heart attack in his Hawaiian condo. Forced relaxation almost killed him.

The second case concerns a hard-driving but somewhat phlegmatic businessman who never dealt with his feelings. At age fifty-five, Sol suffered a heart attack, but that was only the beginning of his problems. His daughter urged him to sell his business and retire to Florida. Not knowing enough about himself or what would make him healthy, he was convinced by her pleadings and agreed to retire. But in Florida, he was miserable, having lost a sense of meaning and control over his life. His health gradually deteriorated, and he suffered for many years from a series of degenerative diseases. Such examples serve to illustrate the findings of controlled scientific research.

The importance of considering individual personality in promoting health was first brought home to me almost a decade ago when I lectured to a large group of medical personnel on the role of emotions in physical health. In part of my talk, I explained that all Type A characteristics were not unhealthy and that there were many people who did just fine being energetic, active, and hardworking. After the talk, a psychiatrist rushed up to me and told me how he was just then applying this idea to the treatment of a very hardworking, competitive, and stressed man. Efforts to teach this wealthy but sickly man to slow down and relax had failed miserably, but this insightful and resourceful psychiatrist had succeeded in helping this patient by funneling his high energy into more positive directions. The man was directed toward using his extensive business experience to aid small businesses trying to get established in his hometown. The patient was still active and hardworking but was no longer stressed. He felt reborn. Distress had been turned into *eustress*—the good stress of interesting challenge. It would, of course, have been a big mistake to force this active, dominant patient to become more restrained and inhibited.

WHAT WORKS?

When a person develops a healing emotional style, you can literally see the difference. The person's nonverbal expressions become more healthy looking. The melancholic's voice becomes louder, his gaze becomes more direct, and his gestures become more animated. The choleric's body tension relaxes, his posture opens up, and his facial expressions become less threatening. The phlegmatic's expressions become more emotionally revealing, her gestures become more dominant, and her speech becomes more emphatic. We may not recognize why, but we find self-healing people to be more likable.

I was skeptical and intrigued when I analyzed my first laboratory findings and found that a person's health could reliably be judged by naive observers who were looking at videotapes or listening to audiotapes. With further study, I recognized that my untrained observers were merely doing (admittedly imperfectly) what experienced clinicians have been doing for a long time—diagnosing health in part from nonverbal cues. This is not magic; rather, it is a systematic evaluation of valid indicators of emotional health, psychophysiological motivation, and vigor. I remember the time fifteen years ago when my own personal physician took one look at me as I staggered into his office and said, "You either have mono or hepatitis." It was indeed mononucleosis, the result of a yearlong series of stressful events.

But just as we cannot simply will our way to health, we also cannot directly change our nonverbal emotional styles. Instead, long-term, gradual interventions must be instituted. When Gerald Ford suddenly became president of the United States, he was given instruction by media consultants in how to appear more "presidential." The problem was that people trusted him but were not inspired by him. However, his newly learned gesturing seemed forced and artificial and made the new president appear even less inspiring. It was only after Mr. Ford had been president for a while that his growing inner confidence began to be revealed in his nonverbal style.

Which interventions work? The key to changing a toxic emotional response into a stable healing system involves doing two things: slowly changing habits and selectively altering social environments. When we start doing things in different ways and in different environments, then our personalities change in a corresponding manner. These changes are relatively stable; there is little relapse.

Most usual healthy behaviors do not require much conscious effort. We brush our teeth out of habit, we wash our hands out of habit, and we protect ourselves from bad weather without extensive thought. (These activities are not natural, they are learned; children or the mentally impaired may do none of these things.) Some of us also are in the habit of buckling our seat belts, eating a fairly balanced diet, flossing our teeth, and so on. We do not have to decide to do these things each day. We do them more or less automatically. This same approach can be applied to our emotions. There are unhealthy habits of social and emotional responding and there are healthy habits of emotional balance.

Some people with cancer are now in the habit of telling a bedtime story to their children or grandchildren each night, of going to a community discussion group each week, or of attending church every Sunday. They have regular habits of positive social interactions. Some workers with heart disease now read a book for twenty minutes every day during their lunch hour, or listen to classical music during their commute to work, or make concise lists of their weekly goals and accomplishments. They have developed regular habits of coping with intrusive, stressful thoughts in ways that are appropriate for them. They were not born knowing how to do these things; they gradually learned how to develop a healing personality. It would have been better, of course, if they had done so before they became ill.

Some people with arthritis or with migraines have cultivated new habits of exercising every morning or stopping at the health club on the way home from work. Some prefer to go for a walk and then climb into a hot tub. Others make sure to meditate every other day. They have developed healthy habits of physical fitness. Again, the important point is that these are all *habits*. They are likely to be followed because they have become a part of everyday living. Fortunately, there are easily learned strategies and tactics that help the self-healing person maintain these good emotional habits.

Other people also have very strong habits, but they are unhealthy ones. The common misdeeds are easy to recognize. Cholerics may honk their horns and fret about the road conditions while driving to work; returning home, they quarrel with their spouses. Melancholics may avoid community groups, watch a lot of television, or engage in self-pity. Phlegmatics may procrastinate in tending to their personal affairs or succumb apathetically to the demands of those around them. These people have poor coping habits that can change for the better, at little cost.

As with any habit, practice makes perfect. The more we do something a certain way, the more likely we are to continue doing it that way. Interestingly, often the reason we get started down a certain path is obscure or even random. Why does one choleric man interrupt others in conversation and then sit sullenly as he is excluded from the group? The most relevant reason is that he has always done so. If we can learn the secrets to doing things a different way, then new habits can form.

This chapter explains many of the ways to change daily routines to promote a healing personality. But habit is only half the equation. Complementary and equally important is social environment. What exactly is "social environment"?

When I was a graduate student, I sometimes ate dinner at the Harvard Law School. Mounted on a wall in the large dining room was a television. Many students watched the evening news during dinner. But what really caught the attention of the law students was the following program, reruns of the *Perry Mason* show. Perry Mason was of course a trial lawyer, and the law students enjoyed seeing how lawyers behave.

Lawyers dress relatively alike. At the least, it is easy to distinguish a group of lawyers from a group of physicians or a group of professors. Each group has similarities in dress, grooming, and accessories. They also have a shared language and, more often than not, shared interests.

By deciding to become a lawyer, a person sets himself or herself up to become similar to other lawyers. Of course, there are many significant differences among lawyers, but there are more similarities. Our personal habits and identities depend to a large extent on the groups with which we associate.

What this conclusion means is that we have some control over the type of person we will be, at least over the long term. If we simply say, "Today, I'm going to start acting as ethically as a minister," then we are unlikely to succeed. But if we *become* a minister (or even a lay minister), then we are more likely to behave ethically than we would if we joined a profession that attracts less idealistic members.

Obviously, it is not feasible for most people to keep switching careers in order to change their personalities. But one *can* switch friends, clubs, housing, neighborhoods, schools, hobbies, volunteer settings, churches, and many other groups that influence personality.

Individuals can shift to associations that fit their predispositions and that lead to a more balanced life-style. For example, one irrepressible young man did wonders for his headaches when he switched from a beer-guzzling bowling team to a health-crazed vegetarian jogging society. For a reticent arthritis patient, a switch from nightly television viewing to volunteer service at a local charity did the trick. For others, a radical switch such as a move to a new career in a different city may work, but such dramatic changes are risky and usually are not necessary. In almost all cases, as social affiliations change, there will be a corresponding change in personality.

For people with a serious chronic illness, such as cancer, a special sort of help is very beneficial. When Terese Lasser had a mastectomy for breast cancer, she stumbled across the idea of the best help of all. She founded Reach to Recovery, an organization that provides help and encouragement to mastectomy patients. Perhaps more important, as Lasser discovered, reaching out to help others who are similarly afflicted is one of the best ways to help oneself!

Why are traditional medical approaches to promoting a healing personality often so incomplete? As we have seen, treatment is far too often directed by a conceptually inadequate medical model that cannot truly integrate the full range of influences on health. Organizations like Reach to Recovery are generally seen as "ancillary" ("secondary") care in a hospital. The hospital's emphasis is on stamping out disease, not on bolstering health. However, as our understanding of the healing personality increases, we become better and better able to devise helpful interventions.

TOO BUSY?

I've never heard people say that they were too busy to watch the Superbowl or the seventh game of the World Series. In fact, if you go out on the highways or visit popular stores during such games (as I have done), you will find them almost deserted. Everyone is home watching TV.

Few people die because they did not have enough time to eat. Sure, we may miss a meal now and then, but eventually we will stop our other activities in order to eat. Similarly, no one has ever died of lack of sleep.

The obvious point of this discussion is that people make time to do those things they most want to do. The excuse that they cannot exercise or socialize or relax because they do not have enough time is phony. The real problem is that many people do not know how to make the time to take care of themselves. And when they do make the time, they don't know how to *maintain* the healthful activities.

One problem concerns what psychologists call delayed gratification. Many people do not have time for the important things because they cannot put off immediate self-indulging activities. For example, one athletically inclined man had trouble getting out to his club to exercise because he loved to read the newspaper from cover to cover upon returning home from work. By then it was "too late" and he was "too tired" to exercise. His solution was to read the newspaper in his health club lounge *after* a period of vigorous exercise.

I have never seen a heart attack victim, who is experiencing crushing chest pain and is in critical condition, decide to check out of the hospital and go back to work. What good is finishing some unfinished business if it is probable that you will die in the process? Yet *before* the heart attack, many people are very willing to engage in a variety of behaviors that are likely to kill them.

In short, although the first step in developing a healing personality is to determine which social environments are best for a particular individual, the second step is to give top priority to the needed changes. The third step is to make the necessary basic changes in one's daily routines.

SCIENCE AND NEW AGE HOLISTIC HEALING

My first encounter with Dr. Dean Ornish was a memorable one. It occurred about a decade ago in the middle of a cold Boston winter. Dr. Ornish was a medical fellow at Harvard and I was a visiting scholar. I learned of his interest in health promotion through my sister, a friend of his. I called him to discuss some new ideas about psychology and health. I left a telephone message.

Half an hour later Dr. Ornish called back, and I launched into an exposition of my new ideas and plans about health research. After about five minutes Dr. Ornish interrupted me. "It sounds very interesting," he said, "but I'm standing in the rain at a public telephone. Could we talk again later?" He had received my message through his electronic pager and had pulled his car over as soon as he had found a phone. I was very embarrassed.

If Dr. Ornish is a Type A man, in the sense of being extremely conscientious and hardworking, he probably is one of the healthy Type As. Trying to develop a comprehensive new approach to healing heart disease, Dr. Ornish moved west and began a major study of psychosocial and behavioral influences on the atherosclerotic process. This study is indeed finding some remarkable success in reversing plaque buildup. Clogged arteries can sometimes be cleaned out without drugs or a surgeon's knife. Sometimes changes in diet, stress management, and life-style can do the trick.

This story of Dr. Ornish is intended to illustrate two points. First, the scientific application of psychosocial interventions to promoting health is a very recent phenomenon. A decade ago, those of us interested in health psychology were excitedly searching the country for like-minded colleagues who would talk about new proposals concerning the nature of health and healing. The second point is that radical but extremely well-credentialed and hardworking thinkers like Dr. Ornish are slowly but surely making their way into the medical establishment. Medical care is starting to change.

Most people have heard about holistic healing and so-called New Age living. In my opinion, such terms refer to cultural movements that have some fine and some not-so-fine components. The good side of such movements is that they redress the overly technical, narrow approach of traditional medicine. The harmful side is that they sometimes take on a cultlike aura or a missionary zeal. In this book, I am not preaching a new religion. Rather, I am presenting the results of the scientific research of myself and others, and I am drawing out what I see to be the implications of this research. We must proceed carefully and scientifically, but we should not ignore the mass of findings rapidly accumulating regarding the healing personality.

In the well-conducted, long-term Western Electric study of depression and cancer, it was found that the relationship between depression and cancer became weaker as the decades progressed. Similarly, the well-done, long-term Western Collaborative Group study of Type A characteristics and heart attacks has found that the significant relationship between Type A and heart attacks diminishes twenty or so years later. To me, such findings are good news. They mean that people can slowly change their personalities over time and thus reduce their risks, just as cigarette smokers can reduce their risks by quitting.

The techniques that are effective for reversing some disease processes and for promoting good health are multifaceted. The public is most likely to hear about dietary changes, at least partly because food companies can make (or lose) large profits as the eating habits of millions change. (I noticed that the promotion and price of oatmeal jumped as soon as news of its cholesterol-lowering effects appeared.) Proper diet is indeed important. However, techniques of stress management—ways to maintain psychosocial equilibrium—are equally important.

Scientists are uncomfortable making recommendations. There is always more evidence to be gathered. There will always be new qualifications on existing recommendations. There is the possibility of unforeseen consequences of a recommendation. Yet consumers are not waiting for the final answer; they are acting every day. I think they are often acting on fragmentary advice and should be considering the *larger picture*. The rest of this chapter presents my distillation of practical tips from the most recent of my colleagues' and my research.

Although I welcome the efforts of all researchers in this field, I have two quarrels with some of my colleagues. First, I believe that much study and advice is too narrowly focused. Work about "how to heal your heart through meditation" is inadequate and even misleading if it fails to consider the many other aspects of and influences on health. Some people get little or no benefit from meditation, and anyway, what good is a healthy heart if the rest of your body has fallen apart? Second, I believe that much previous work fails to consider the overall environmental context in which individuals live.

MORE BALANCE

"For all deaths, there was a U-shaped relation to the serum cholesterol level." This statement is typical scientific jargon from a leading medical journal. But it has a remarkable translation. It means that in one recent large-scale study of 350,000 men, those with abnormally high *or* abnormally low levels of cholesterol in their blood were more likely to die. Men with average levels were more likely to live.

If you dig deeply, you will find such relationships in many scientific studies. They are not highlighted in the scientific reports and they are not trumpeted in newspaper headlines. Such "U-shaped" relations are not appealing, especially to Americans; they mean one can have too much of a good thing—too much exercise, too much dieting, or too much medication. When the body's internal environment shows signs of imbalance—too much or too little of something—the risk of illness rises. Just how much is too much or too little differs from person to person.

So, are we back with the timeless wisdom "Everything in moderation"? Not really, because "moderation," too, varies from person to person and situation to situation. Better advice is "To thine own self be true." But we now know much more about what it means to be balanced and true. And we know a lot more about *how* to achieve this balance.

My research has made it clear to me that the development and progression of common chronic diseases sometimes can be affected by efforts to restore internal balance. Some conditions are influenced more easily than others, and some people are affected more than others. In my opinion, however, it is just as much a mistake to assume that psychological and social interventions are not important to health as it is to assume that biological factors are not important to health.

Internal balance depends in part on external balance. If you tend to be depressed or apathetic, then you should not be undertaking the kinds of changes that would be more appropriate for someone who is mostly hostile and angry. And vice versa. In this chapter, I first include an explanation of how to ascertain the demands of the social environment and how to determine the degree of mismatch between personality and environment. I then take up the final step—how to institute changes so that one can have the right habits in the right environments.

In sum, the existing evidence suggests that the techniques described in this chapter will not only help prevent disease but also will help prevent the progression of chronic diseases, especially if the techniques are tailored to the individual. Such interventions are not miracle cures—they should not be used to interrupt ongoing medical treatment. The psychological and social implications of any treatments and medications should be discussed with one's own physician.

WAYS OF HEALING

A tremendous challenge facing many older Americans is the need for surgery or other invasive medical care. Work initiated during the 1950s shows that patients vary greatly before and after surgery. Before surgery, some patients worry dreadfully about their operations and feel very vulnerable. Other patients are somewhat concerned and ask for information about their surgery. Still other patients are extremely cheerful and relaxed before their operations and do not want to know about the medical details.

Which patients heal best? After surgery, the patients who were highly fearful *as well as* the totally fearless patients generally experience relatively poor postoperative reactions; those patients with a moderate amount of anticipatory fear recover best. That is, not only is it not good to be too pessimistic, it also is not good to be excessively optimistic. This conclusion goes contrary to the overly simple assertion that optimistic people are healthier.

Mental rehearsal of solutions to realistic problems, a moderate level of anticipatory fear, and a preparatory working through of difficulties helps patients deal with the stresses of medical procedures. Patients who are excessively optimistic may be shocked by the pain and challenge of recovery and may be denying their hidden fears. They also may have trouble turning to others for help, since they have asserted that everything is fine. Furthermore, patients who are unrealistic in their expectations about illness may be less willing to work on improving their overall physical condition, both before and after surgery. In medical battles, as in wartime battles, it is not adaptive to be terrified, but it is not helpful to be cocky and overconfident, either.

An intriguing example of this phenomenon comes from a study conducted on male heart patients in a San Diego hospital who were awaiting coronary bypass surgery. Some of the patients were placed with a hospital roommate who was already recovering from surgery. Others had a roommate who was likewise awaiting surgery. Although the patients placed with a recovering patient were able to see the pain and problems of postsurgical recovery, they actually became less anxious about their own surgery. Most important, the patients who had been waiting with a recovering patient were found to be more likely to have a better recovery from their own surgery. They were more likely to be active after their own surgery and were released from the hospital sooner than bypass patients who had waited with presurgery patients.

Yale psychologist Irving Janis, who first began this line of research, gives the following example. A young woman underwent an appendectomy and had no problems afterward. She had been moderately worried beforehand but had discussed her worries, and she recovered beautifully. A few years later, she returned to the same hospital for another abdominal surgery—removal of her gall bladder. Her physician assured her, "There's really nothing to it." She did not worry at all. After the operation, when she encountered the usual but unexpected pains and privations, she became markedly upset and negativistic, angry at her doctor. Again in this case, it may be common sense that it's best not to worry, but the common sense is wrong!

The example of recovery from surgery points out that there are several types of influences on healing. First, there are marked differences in how people think about stress. Patients can be excessively anxious, blissfully ignorant, or mentally prepared and realistic. Second, there are differences in how patients relate to other people. Interactions in a hospital room can be depressing, pitying, dishonest, and pessimistic, or they can be encouraging, relieving, open, and soothing. Third, there are differences in the physical steps people take in response to stress and illness. A surgical patient could be passively monitored and left to rest and recuperate, or the patient could be gotten up and about, with things to do to relieve discomfort and decisions to make about treatment. Let us put this all together.

A challenging event is not necessarily stressful unless the individual interprets it as excessively dangerous. Thus, *psychological coping* involves efforts at controlling interpretations and thought processes. A person can learn to think in certain ways in order to make the stressful life event less important or less traumatizing. Part of developing a self-healing personality involves learning the ways these psychic reappraisals can be encouraged; we can learn to think in ways that relieve stress.

The second major source of adaptive coping comes from *social relations*. When faced with life changes and the resulting stress, self-healing personalities know how to gather the support of spouses and friends as a significant aid to coping. For example, on average, married people are much healthier than divorced or widowed people. The difference is due partly to the stress of losing one's partner, but it also is true that single people generally have a more difficult time dealing with environmental stressors. The loss of other social ties has a similar detrimental effect.

A striking example of social loss is provided by sociologist Kai Erikson, who studied the effects of a terrible flood in the mountain town of Buffalo Creek, West Virginia. Social ties and sense of community were destroyed by this flood, and many people subsequently became ill. They felt drained, exhausted, and weak. As Erikson put it, their emotional shelter was stripped away and the community could "no longer enlist its members in a conspiracy to make a perilous world seem safe." Part of this chapter explains how social relations work to improve health and what one can do to improve social support.

Finally, a disease-resistant personality also can be achieved through direct *biological means*. We can learn relevant activities that encourage a different physiological reaction in the individual from the usual stress responses. Behaviors such as exercise, systematic relaxation, and meditation are appropriate for particular individuals, although meditation is not for everyone.

Men and women in their forties often ask me whether jogging is healthy. Physical exercise can indeed help some people cope effectively with stress, through several different processes, though not always the processes they expect. Most simply, going outdoors to run can serve to remove a person from the stimuli that cause stress—such as work pressures at the office or family pressures at home. Second, focusing on one's body, breathing, and bodily sensations with repetitive movements may serve to invoke the body's natural relaxation responses. Finally, direct physiological responses will occur in some people. "Runner's high"—a feeling of euphoria felt during exercise—seems to be caused by physiological factors involving the changed metabolism. Each of these processes may be appropriate for certain people in certain situations.

In short, there are many devices that disease-resistant people use to deal with the stresses of a challenging world. Gurus are not necessary; with some dedicated effort, almost anyone can learn simple techniques best suited to them. These techniques are especially effective for ordinary people facing the usual stresses of our time; they are not effective for people with serious mental illness.

EMOTIONAL PROBLEMS

The Individual

One way to have emotional imbalance diagnosed is to seek professional advice. This is a good idea if one seems unable to function in daily life. (Serious problems include inability to hold a job, being stuck in an abusive relationship, extreme fears that limit activity, severe depression with suicidal thoughts, and so on.) But most people do not need professional help to develop a healing personality.

It is necessary first to evaluate oneself as an individual to determine one's usual patterns of emotional responding. How can this be done? First, one can evaluate oneself on the symptoms reviewed below. Next, one can collect the evaluation of a spouse or a sibling. And third, a close friend can be asked to make the evaluation. If there is agreement, then you probably are being accurate about your usual emotional state.

Let us briefly review the common emotional reaction patterns and discuss their symptoms and appearances.

Melancholic

People with melancholic emotional patterns are, of course, more predisposed to cry than most people. They may think about death or the end of the world. They are often (but not constantly) down in the dumps and sometimes mope along in a dispirited manner. There are other common but less-often recognized symptoms. Melancholics may sleep too little, arising with a start very early in the morning. Or they may sleep too much and generally feel weak and tired. They may have a diminished appetite and sexual desire.

The chronically melancholic feel little hope of overcoming challenges. They may lose some of their ability to concentrate. They generally give up easily and circumvent hurdles. They often speak softly and move languidly. They are more likely to be women than men.

Phlegmatic

Some superficially similar symptoms also characterize apathy. Phlegmatic or apathetic people often are subordinate and weak, but they do not profess sadness. In fact, they may try to appear friendly.

They are calm, but *too* calm—not much excites them to action. They have little real curiosity and may avoid interacting with other people. They have few realistic plans or explicit ambitions. They have little sense of internal control; they drift along with the flow of events. They are inactive, but they may have occasional outbursts of feeling. As with melancholic people, the apathetic have low self-esteem. Both depressed and apathetic people often have many minor physical aches and pains. They may take a lot of aspirin or other analgesics.

Phlegmatic people may appear nervous. They are generally submissive and tense. They often have protectively crossed legs and a closed body position. They have many acquaintances but few real friends.

Choleric

Hostile people are, of course, angry much of the time. They have tense faces and stiff but emphatic bodies. They are easily excitable. They are often very active. They seem to have a chip on their shoulders—a kind of bitterness toward the world. They find many situations frustrating. They may be sarcastic and moody.

Cholerics are dominant but not especially likable. They may make many posture shifts and nervous arm and leg movements. They respond aggressively when challenged.

Sanguine

Enthusiastic or sanguine people infect others with their exuberance. They are not ecstatic but rather are generally responsive and content. Often they also are active and energetic, although some are calm and self-assured. They are alert, curious, secure, and constructive.

Sanguines generally enjoy being around other people and have close friends. In social interaction, sanguines smile naturally and maintain eye contact. They have smooth gestures and often talk rapidly. They feel in control.

Everyone has some of these characteristics some of the time. And everyone has some basic predispositions. But to the extent that people can move from the imbalances of melancholy, apathy, and hostility toward the balance of the sanguine, the less stress they will experience and the healthier they will become.

The next step in the self-assessment process is to determine one's strengths and weaknesses. That is, which aspects of ourselves bring out these emotional states? What can we do well and not so well, and what are our relevant likes and dislikes?

A good way to make these evaluations systematically is to use the following five dimensions: Are you more extroverted and outgoing, or are you an introverted and solitary type of person? Are you more impulsive and unsocialized, or careful and calculating? Are you more active or more easygoing? Are you more intellectual or more of a hands-on person? And finally, are you more emotional or more rational? Again, these evaluations should be made by you, by a spouse or sibling, and by a close friend.

Once these characteristics have been determined, we need to determine how our personalities fit with our environments. The mismatch of personal characteristics and environments produce the emotional imbalances. We thus face the difficult task of evaluating our usual situations and environments.

The Situation

The situation is too often ignored. We have many terms for and much experience in describing our personalities and our emotional reactions, but usually we do not carefully evaluate our situations. Yet it is often the social situation that is the source of the problem. Even though we have some personality problems, we may do just fine in the right environments.

Contrary to what many books and articles assert, modern society is not necessarily stressful. Many people thrive in a large urban environment and others are miserable down on the farm. Why do some people react poorly to the rapid changes of modern society?

As outlined in previous chapters, there are two main sources of problems. First, it is generally not a good idea to be in an uncontrollable situation. Second, and more important, it is generally a bad idea to be in a situation that does not fit your personality. With such a mismatch—for example, a calm, easygoing person working as a firefighter; or an impulsive, emotional person working as a physician; or an introverted, intellectual person working as a salesperson—there is likely to be a resulting harmful emotional reaction: depression, hostility, or apathy.

The classic example of a harmful mismatch is to put an active, self-confident elderly person into a traditional, regimented nursing home. It is well documented that the negative emotions that result lead inexorably to physical decline. On the other hand, if a somewhat timid and lonely octogenarian moves from an ancient, isolated apartment into an appropriately structured retirement community, health may improve rapidly. Are retirement homes good or bad? It depends on the person as well as on the home. Well-meaning social activists who denounce retirement homes are just as wrong as well-meaning health care professionals who assert that for their own good, all old, weak individuals should be institutionalized.

I remember one case in which a proud, independent old man was placed into a retirement home that focused on group activities, including day trips to museums and in-house recreational plays and shows. His son had read that social interaction was good for old folks. The old man was miserable without his solitude and time for reflection; he finally had to be moved to a different setting. Although it is true that positive social relations are generally healthful, it was a mistake to ignore the mismatch between the individual's orientation and the group's goals.

For working adults, the easiest way to characterize common environments is to do so in terms of jobs and careers. This is where we spend the most time, and it is where the most demands are made on us. Two important and very relevant job characteristics are the pace of work and the amount of individual control that is allowed. The following is a rough guide to classifying work environments.

Generally speaking, the following types of positions are relatively slow paced and controllable: computer programmer, civil engineer, writer, artist, appliance repairperson, truck driver. These jobs can be quite demanding, but the minute-to-minute pace is less often a hurried one. (Of course, a nasty boss could alter the relative independence of such jobs.) This is not the place for an active, impulsive person—it is not hard to find a miserable computer programmer (with ulcers) who really wanted a career involving professional sports. Another very common job that is still even paced and controllable but is especially extroverted and emotional is that of independent salesperson—perfect for an easygoing, sociable, and friendly kind of individual.

The following positions generally are slow paced and *un*controllable: janitor, security guard, farm laborer, bus driver. There is a fixed, controlled routine. These posts generally bring at least some stress (due to the uncontrollability), but they are especially stressful if there is a conflict with a basic dimension of one's personality. For example, in one case involving two brothers with jobs in these categories, the docile, unmotivated younger brother was quite content and healthy, while his ambitious older sibling lived a bitter life with chest pain.

Examples of fast-paced and generally controllable professions are: physician (private practice), business executive, supervisor, police officer. Put a slow-paced, relaxed person in such a position and a helpless, phlegmatic emotional state may result—as in the case of an introverted, calculating, easygoing young woman who became a physician because her father told her that librarians did not earn enough money. She became more and more withdrawn and repressed until she suddenly picked herself up and moved to Maine, setting up a small rural practice. Contrary to common expectation, fast-paced positions may not be stressful at all if they are filled by the right kinds of people. Many a successful businessman grew up as an ambitious, unsocialized brat, waiting for a chance to make his mark.

Fast-paced and uncontrollable professions: waiter, cashier, assembler, air traffic controller, firefighter, nurse. These jobs are generally the most stressful, but they are especially bad for an easygoing, rational, and calculating type of person. Other people, active but without clear long-term goals, thrive in these positions, with no health problems whatsoever.

Careers also can be classified on dimensions of intellectual demands, level of physical activity, and degree of emotional creativity involved. Indeed, sometimes there is a significant mismatch on these other dimensions—as in the case of an aspiring writer who takes a job as a waitress. But usually the important mismatches are on the dimensions of pace and control.

In extreme cases, the ideal solution to a mismatch problem is to switch jobs. But often that solution is neither practical nor healthy. Most people cannot walk away from their professions, their businesses, their families (for homemakers), and so on. In most cases, the realistic solution involves learning to deal with or cope with the current pressures. Fortunately, learning to cope is very possible, and the rest of this chapter explains how.

Another way of thinking about the demands of the situation or environment is in terms of the major tasks or challenges in life that one currently is facing. A person can evaluate whether his or her resources are the right ones for the tasks ahead. For example, getting married is a major change in one's life and may be (but is not necessarily) stressful. Starting a career involves a very demanding series of adaptations, and sometimes that is traumatic. Retiring from work eliminates a series of demands but introduces a whole new series of challenges which may or may not be successfully faced. Of course, moving to a new city, marital separation, pregnancy and childbirth, and financial setbacks also are especially challenging times, each with its own unique set of demands. Less commonly thought of in these terms but extremely challenging nonetheless is the fighting of a chronic illness.

Problems can arise in several ways. There can be conflicts between different goals. A typical example is that of a woman who wants to advance in her career and raise a family. Each environment is demanding, and the demands conflict. But aside from the objective demands, the distress arises in part as a function of how the woman thinks about herself, the quality of her relations with others, and her biological coping techniques.

Second, people may be unsure about their suitability for the tasks—they may not really want to succeed. People with low self-esteem or phlegmatics with "big eyes" but repressed feelings can easily become trapped in situations that produce more and more stress.

Third, there may simply be a lack of ability to meet the demands of the situation. I know physicians who are miserable because they cannot cope with dying patients, professors who suffer because they cannot bring themselves to write regularly, salespersons who are nervous at meeting people, and clergy who lose interest in their parishioners' problems.

In sum, it is helpful to have a good understanding of the nature of the directly relevant causes of stress in order to make the best possible effort to cope. But now let us turn directly to the coping techniques themselves.

THINKING ABOUT STRESS: CHANGING THOUGHTS

A fundamental insight of clinical psychology can be very helpful to most people suffering from stress. If you go to a good therapist and say, "My lover is dreadfully inconsiderate and ignores my complaints," most likely the therapist will respond, "And how does that make you feel?" What the psychotherapist understands is that we have relatively little power to directly affect the behaviors of others, but we have enormous power to alter our own reactions and interpretations. The psychological insight is: we waste too much time trying to change other people, when we should be changing ourselves.

Ironically, it is often the case that when we change ourselves, the behaviors of others will change as well.

Thus, the first major method of coping is to change how we think about the challenges we face. However, I have already argued that we cannot do this directly. What can we do?

Success Reminders

When my young son accomplishes a small task, such as climbing over an obstacle, he lets out a gleeful cry of self-satisfaction. He has succeeded. When a woman with arthritis manages to cook a gourmet meal or draw a fine picture in the art class she teaches, she similarly reacts with positive, healing emotions. A good day.

We all need concrete reminders that we are successful, competent people. If we structure our days and weeks so that we have some good chances to accomplish things (even small things) of merit, we will build self-regard. On the other hand, if the arthritic patient visits the concert hall only to lament that she no longer can perform a Mozart piano concerto, her other thoughts also will tend to turn negative.

One troubled woman with phlegmatic tendencies managed to keep herself stable through the technique of making lists—lists of goals and lists of things to do. A key to the successful use of lists is to *mix* easy and difficult tasks. A weekly list that includes such simple items as "Call John to thank him for his help" and "Buy Bellow's new novel" as well as the more difficult "Do income taxes" and "Repaint kitchen" makes challenges seem more manageable and gives us the satisfaction (morale boost) of being able to check off items as we complete them.

Lists also serve the purpose of improving the efficiency of time use. This is especially important for cholerics, who tend to be worried about time. There is nothing unhealthy about having a full schedule, so long as the important tasks are all on the list. It is surprising to me to see the number of hardworking, competitive people who forget or ignore important events or activities and later pay the consequences in emotional disruptions.

Benjamin Franklin used the technique of success reminders centuries before any psychologist walked the earth. He proceeded as follows. First he made a list of thirteen virtuous goals, such as temperance ("Eat not to dullness"), order ("Let all things have their place; let each part of business have its time"), moderation ("Avoid extremes"), and industry ("Be always employed in something useful"). He then constructed a little calendar book, with rows of the virtues and columns of the days of week. He focused on one virtue each week, and at the end of each day would put a black mark on his chart if he had violated the virtue that day. In this way, Franklin gradually minimized his bad habits, thus creating a clean slate.

Self-rewards must be designed and virtues chosen with one's personality in mind. Melancholics need to reward their senses of competence, persistence, and optimism. For them, setting out a structured program of small steps toward a goal is useful. For example, one distressed cancer patient laid out a yearlong series of activities to help the development of her children. She then coped well with her illness.

Phlegmatics should attend to issues of activity, friendship, and control. One forty-five-year-old phlegmatic succeeded marvelously by becoming a part-time tutor of high school students. A regular routine that encourages close personal interaction (preferably exciting rather than boring) can enhance the phlegmatic's self-perception.

Many phlegmatics also are helped by a long-term life plan evaluation. A simple exercise is to write down an outline of one's biography and then project into the future—five years, ten years, fifteen years. This exercise may be impetus for a phlegmatic to see that it is time *right now* to leave a dead-end relationship or go back to school or join a church activities club.

Cholerics can choose goals that will encourage feelings of relaxation and cooperation. Planning enjoyable social activities on a regular basis may be helpful. One business executive began giving monthly parties for small groups of his employees, an activity he hated at first but soon came to enjoy. Social success led to changed perceptions of the business environment.

Sometimes it helps to try to identify patterns of unhealthy negative feelings. One woman found that she felt butterflies in her stomach and pains in her chest whenever she had to make telephone calls. Upon reflection, this seemed to be a pattern that had continued since some unpleasant experiences during her teenage years. In this case, then, the trick was to make a series of gradually more difficult telephone calls one weekend and to keep track of her increasing success.

Self-esteem

At my college graduation dinner, actress Shirley MacLaine was the featured speaker. She urged us to "be free" and fulfill our potential. Although her speech was reasonable and well intentioned, it was not well received. However noble the thoughts, many people have trouble responding to advice to think positive, appreciate each day, and so on. Such advice is sometimes perceived as trite, banal, hackneyed. Today is the first day of the rest of your life, but that is upsetting if you are disappointed with your life.

There are several proven ways to improve one's self-esteem, the best being to receive feedback from others that you have done something worthwhile. If I receive a letter from a respected colleague praising one of my books or scientific articles, I tend to feel terrific for the next couple of days. It is not only that I have received some praise, but also that I appreciate the praise. A melancholic may reject the praise; a choleric may ignore it. So at least some of the praise must be clear and forceful.

Charities and other volunteer organizations recognize the importance of forceful praise. It is not enough to merely thank their volunteers and donors. Rather, they must throw dinners and tributes in which the depth of appreciation is made crystal clear. The volunteers and donors, in turn, feel good about themselves and continue their efforts. Almost everyone has something that they do well or that is valuable to others, and it is a straightforward though not always easy step to continue to do it. Yet often people are urged to give up their favorite hobbies—"You're always working on the car." "You always want to play bridge." "You only care about the theater; why don't we ever go camping?" This is another example of how so-called common-sense advice from others can be bad advice.

How can we respond to such unhealthy advice? Recognize that usually the complaint is not really about the hobby, it is about feelings of abandonment. That is, ignore the content but address the feelings. If things have not gotten too far out of hand, a simple solution is to reply, "I enjoy working on my car; it relaxes and refreshes me. Why don't we plan some time right now to do something that you like to do?"

For phlegmatics, another good but simple means of improving self-esteem is to write a narrative of the situational constraints on one's life and one's good traits in reaction to these challenges. For example, a young runner with migraines wrote a story about his athletic success, despite occasional pain and incapacitation. Looking over the narrative, you may find that you are not such a distressed person after all. An alternative way to approach this issue is to write one's own obituary, emphasizing (as do real obituaries) one's positive qualities. This approach is good for phlegmatics, since it helps them get in touch with their feelings. It is less useful for melancholics, who may overemphasize their negative qualities.

A further way to improve self-esteem is to associate, even indirectly, with someone who values our talents. For many people, this can be an inspiring minister, such as Billy Graham, Norman Vincent Peale, or Robert Schuller. For others, it can be an optimistic and inspiring community leader. For still others, it is simply a group of friends who like and appreciate you.

Visual Imagery

A number of years ago, I took a course on psychosocial issues in coping with cancer. It was attended mostly by nurses who worked on the cancer wards. One day, one of the speakers launched into a description of the "blue light" that emanates from the center of the earth and appears in the room of every cancer patient when the room lights are turned off. The speaker advised the class to teach patients to raise their internal antennas to pick up this blue light. It would bring peace and healing.

After this presentation, I raised my hand and raised an objection. Sure, I knew that healing was facilitated by faith. I knew all about the placebo effect and its benefits for the chronically ill. But wasn't this pseudo-scientific mumbo jumbo about a blue light a little much?

To my shock and amazement, some of the nurses in the class stood up to defend the speaker. They thought it was a wonderful insight, and they were going to teach their patients to raise their internal antennas toward the blue light.

As the discussion went on, it dawned on me that some of these nurses were under extreme stress. They had to deal with and treat the emotions of desperate cancer patients, but the doctors in particular and the medical care system in general gave them absolutely no guidance or support. Here, however, this speaker was offering specific advice about what could be done.

Fortunately, today most nurses, social workers, and others who deal constantly with the feelings of the chronically ill know all about the technique that has come to be called visualization. Visualization is the imagination of scenes and visions that trigger changes in the body's physiological state.

Let me state right off that I am not a visualization fanatic. Why not? First of all, visualization is not appropriate for everyone. It is probably best for phlegmatics, who have unconscious emotional conflicts or tensions that need to be resolved. It probably is not helpful for impatient cholerics, who may conjure up images of battlegrounds and angry competitions. It probably also is not helpful for many melancholics, who may view the blue light as a sign of their impending demise. In a similar way, visits to healing shrines like Lourdes are most likely to help emotionally burned-out phlegmatics who have lost faith and need divine inspiration.

It is almost impossible to prove the scientific validity of visualization. This is because it never occurs in isolation. That is, someone who is "visualizing" regularly also probably is relaxing more, resting more, eating more carefully, and getting along better with friends, family, and physicians. In other words, although visualization often works, we never know exactly why it works. This is not a general indictment of visualization but rather a criticism of its presentation as the royal road to health.

For those who feel they can combat stress through visual imagery and by concentrating on internal conflicts, here is how it is done. First, close your eyes and think about the problem (such as cancer cells growing in one's body). Really concentrate. Then think about a counterbalancing, health-promoting solution. For example, some people imagine themselves floating in clouds, with the stress or the disease being washed away by gentle winds. Others imagine their disease-fighting white blood cells gobbling up cancer cells, sort of like an internal PAC-MAN.

I remember an eminent psychologist describing how he relaxed himself before giving a major address. He knew he would be speaking in a blue room, so he concentrated deeply (actually performing a kind of self-hypnosis) on calm feelings elicited by the color blue. On seeing the blue room, he then felt its calming effect. In other words, a calming thought simply overcame anxious thoughts.

Such a technique can be helpful for people facing stresses at work. If one can practice each night imagining that the workplace makes one feel calm or exhilarated or whatever feeling is most helpful, then it is easier to actually feel this way when entering this work room. Regular practice and deep concentration are essential.

Many people find certain props helpful for visualization. Some people draw pictures of their stresses or diseases. Some write down their dreams upon awakening each morning. Others use guided imagery audiotapes, in which the calm, soothing voice of a therapist instructs you to relax and drift into the clouds. (Don't use these tapes while driving a car!) Still others rely on their favorite music. In each case, the goal is to change how we think about situations that have proven distressing.

Turning Work into Play

"You know, my business is a fun business," said a fit Bob Hope at age eighty, commenting on his longevity. The comedy business is literally a fun business, and yet some humorists are not sanguine but instead have a much darker side. On the other hand, physicians, funeral directors, and others who work in a deadly serious business often develop a healthy sense of humor about their work.

The basic techniques of turning work into play are easy to understand but difficult to implement. For a young child who resists getting dressed or picking up her toys, the clever parent can turn the tasks into a game. I call this the Mary Poppins approach, after the movie character who explained that for every job that must be done there is an element of fun. But can one turn a miserable commute or a nasty boss into a game?

One psychotherapeutic technique that sometimes works is the worst-case scenario. Simply put, one sits in a calm, relaxed setting and imagines the worst that could possibly happen in a bothersome situation. Hate commuting? Imagine that there's a major tie-up on the highway in front of you, your car overheats, your boss is waiting for you to bring him important information, and you need to find a bathroom. So what? Is it the end of the world? Will you still have anything of value in your life? Once the worst case is fully and calmly imagined in all its "horror," the hassles of a traffic commute may not seem so terrible.

Probably the best approach to turning work into play is to develop a sense of humor. I have seen this work for cholerics, phlegmatics, and melancholics. No one knows exactly how to do it, but two procedures work for many people. The first involves a zany, self-conscious attempt at increasing your *perceived* control over your environment. This is basically a giant make-believe game in which you imagine that you can choose not to do your distasteful chores, but that you have decided to do them for your own pleasure! That is, you pretend to be the Marx brothers. Obviously, this mental technique will not work for everyone; some love it, but others think it is ridiculous.

The second procedure for promoting humor in one's life is to associate with humor and humorists. This could involve reading, watching, and listening to humorous books, shows, and tapes. Or it could involve increasing your associations with people who have a good sense of humor. Over time, one's thoughts about the world begin to shift.

Prioritize

As Harvard Business School wouldn't forget to tell you, a key to successful management is to decide what is most important to accomplish. A closely related skill is knowing what to delegate. These tools do not work only for business executives; they can be used by anyone dealing with stress. They are especially helpful to cholerics.

If you do not bother to pay the rent, feed the pets, gas the car, or lock the door, there may be serious consequences. However, if one does not dust the furniture, read the sports page, or open the junk mail, then there will be more time for the important activities.

For some people, their stress level is greatly reduced when they sit down and decide what is most important for them to do this day, this month, and this year. Less important things, once recognized, can be put off, delegated to others, or even dropped from consideration. This coping technique is most likely to be helpful to cholerics, who are often frustrated by having too much to do. It is less valuable for melancholics, who feel that they have little control over their lives.

Setting priorities is not so easy as it sounds. Most people can make up a list of what is most important, but they have trouble dealing with the consequences of ignored or delegated tasks. Unwashed dishes, unwatched TV, unreturned phone calls, and unattended meetings may bring complaints from spouses, children, salespeople, coworkers, and others. Yet these overlooked activities may have been correctly sacrificed to achieve more important, higher-priority goals.

Dealing with Creeps

There are a few truly rotten people in our lives. Their hateful actions will arouse some negative feelings, and there is not much we can do about it. Does it matter whether we keep this anger in or let it out? Not really. What matters is whether we keep the anger with us or let it go. Some people do well with an emotional outburst to clear the air, while others do just as well by calmly dismissing the whole episode. Screaming "primal" therapies and low-key "imagination" therapies both work if they remove the anger.

One basic psychological insight can be helpful in this area: Most people who anger or depress us are not truly rotten. Rather, they have emotional problems of their own. They are insecure, hassled, or suffering long-term physical or emotional challenges. Surprisingly, they often respond quite well to a gesture of friendship, even a forced gesture. Successful marriage counselors capitalize on this fact. They break down the usual patterns of revenge and escalation and replace these patterns with gestures of caring and cooperation.

Sometimes, however, people really are trapped with a creep (in technical psychiatric terms, someone with a "personality disorder"). One may have an unfair, nasty boss, an impaired teacher, or a totally self-centered spouse. Such unfortunate people may be trapped in the unhealthy situation of high demands and few personal resources. However, if one is healthy in other ways—that is, has good emotional habits and some good social relationships—then the health effects of the creep may be minimized.

At age seventy, Dr. Jonas Salk, inventor of the polio vaccine, described his secret to staying young: "I keep working at what I like to do and I remain part of the community." A healing personality not only knows how to think positively about life but also recognizes the importance of other people—the importance of community social support.

SOCIAL SUPPORT: CHANGING RELATIONSHIPS

There is a story about a young man who was proud to be learning to ride a horse. He always insisted on riding the largest, most muscular horse in the stables, even though he was really quite a poor horseman. Why did he insist on the largest horse? He believed that he once overheard a high compliment from a female observer who remarked to her friend, "Look at the ass on that horse."

"Social support" is the current jargon for having good relations with other people, especially friends. There is excellent evidence that people with close relationships are better able to resist stress and disease. The self-healing personality gets in touch with inner feelings through close, self-revealing discussion with others. This is especially important for phlegmatics, who repress their feelings, and for cholerics, who tend to be hostile and suspicious toward others. But many people, like the horseman, misinterpret the valuable feedback they receive from others.

If you live in Alameda County, in northern California, you may have been studied by social scientists as part of the most famous study of social support. The seminal part of this study followed thousands of people in the community for almost a decade. As previously noted, the researchers found that people with fewer community ties were more likely to die. This effect was not dependent on preexisting health or economic status.

Japan has a low heart disease rate and high overall longevity statistics. Epidemiologists usually try to explain these observations in terms of the Japanese consumption of fish; fish oils do indeed seem to have some health benefits. But isn't it possible that social support in close-knit Japanese communities could be involved? Perhaps the most provocative study of community social support concerned Japanese-Americans living in California. It was found that those Japanese-Americans who had become acculturated to Western life had a much higher incidence of heart disease than those who had maintained their ethnic and social ties. Other studies have similarly concluded that close social networks lead to better health, as compared to similar groups of people who have lost their close community ties.

How do you know if you have emotional support? One way is to ask yourself the following questions: Is there someone who will listen to me talk about my problems? Is there someone who has faith and confidence in me? (Children do not count.) Is there someone whom I trust and who trusts me? Is there someone who helps me in times of difficulty so that I never feel alone or abandoned?

Obviously, a spouse often will provide good social support. Good marriages are built on healthy self-disclosure. In addition to common sources like a best friend or sibling, it appears that a good resource is a minister or priest. (It is no accident that many people benefit from religious confession.) In a pinch, even a therapist will do. People who can rely on more than one person for support generally are better off than someone with all her eggs in one basket.

Consider the case of Steve, an attorney who has just become a partner in his firm. Steve works sixty to seventy hours a week and enjoys the challenge and the money. His wife is happy to stay at home to care for their daughter. Steve does not smoke and is in good shape. The couple is a member of a large bridge club; they play twice a week. They are also active members of their local synagogue. Steve does not have much time for vacation trips. His wife thinks he works too hard and worries about his health. She buys him self-help books. What should be done? *Prescription:* Steve does not need any interventions to improve his health. His long work week is not a health threat.

Social integration is strongly related, in study after study, to an absence of depression and related forms of mental distress. It is not surprising that good social relations also should be an element of the self-healing personality. It is very risky for one's health to tamper unduly with these relations.

Oftentimes, people who are abandoned by a lover or deceived by a friend make a nice-sounding but dangerous resolution: "I don't need anybody; I can stand on my own two feet." If this means that one will never again be utterly dependent on just one person, then that is fine. If, however, it suggests a general caution and distancing from other people, then it is likely to be unhealthy in the long run. A much better resolution to make at the time of abandonment is: "I don't need *you*; I have lots of other people to turn to."

A caveat is in order here. Social support can be harmful if the particular needs of the patient are not fully considered. For example, a woman with breast cancer who is worried about her physical appearance may be distressed rather than helped if a crowd of well-wishers descends upon her to proclaim blandly that "everything will be perfectly all right—you'll be just as good as new." Specific social ties must be evaluated in terms of their probable impact on the individual.

Getting Social Support

Many people make two big mistakes in seeking social support. First, they look to their jobs—to bosses, coworkers, and business associates. Second, they look to their childhood families—to their parents, their siblings, their aunts and uncles. The problem is that these two sources of support often do not have the necessary compatibility with one's needs.

Few of us choose jobs based primarily on the quality of the people with whom we will be working. Basically, we seek jobs that allow us to use our skills. We also, of course, try to choose jobs that are high paying, reasonably secure, interesting, and near to home. If our co-workers become friends, that is nice; but few people would quit an exciting, secure, high-paying job in pursuit of one that was boring and low paying but had friendlier coworkers. So it should not be surprising that sometimes coworkers are not good sources of social support.

Family members—parents, siblings, cousins—often are easy to reach and sympathetic to our needs. However, although it is nice to know that relatives will always love us, they do not always make the best confidants and friends. They often have their own ideas about what we should be like, and they may become distressed when hearing about our personal problems. Instead, often it is better to seek support from people who truly can share our failings and triumphs.

Consider the case of Jane, a thirty-six-year-old physician in private practice. Jane's marriage fell apart and she has trouble finding dates because of her high professional status. Jane works long hours and has a very high income, but she hates living alone. She often feels somewhat depressed and fears that she will never be able to start a family. She begins to repress her feelings and becomes more and more phlegmatic. Finally she talks over her feelings with a social worker friend. *Prescription:* The friend concludes that Jane should be actively seeking a husband. Jane agrees that finding a suitable husband would open up the possibilities for the life-style she wants. Therefore, she should allocate a large number of hours per week toward meeting new people. Her medical practice should be cut back. She should attend every medical conference in her region and should offer to serve on professional panels. She should attend the two churches in her part of town. And she should exercise daily at the local health club. In short, Jane needs to plan a strong, conscious effort to keep herself physically active and socially available. This plan, which is likely to succeed, may seem obvious once it is laid out. But it is noteworthy how many people do not see the steps they can take to increase their social ties.

Religion

Organized religion has had many problems in adapting ancient theologies and customs to the demands of the modern world. However, our major religions also have evolved to provide a great depth of high-quality social support.

Religion, especially in the United States, has two relevant and appealing aspects. First, it is very easy to join. Basically, all one has to do is show up at a church or temple. Just about all that is needed is a willingness to contribute one's efforts to the community.

The second attraction of local religion is that there are so many to choose from. In any large or even medium-size city, there are congregations and ministers to fit the personal needs and life-styles of almost any individual. A mistake many people make is to give up before they find the congregation that is most suitable for them. Religious organizations are grossly underutilized. Many people could quickly solve their problems of social support if they joined an appropriate religious group.

Not long ago, a proclamation of the "right" way to live, entitled the *Desiderata*, was in popular circulation. Based on biblical sayings, it was attributed to "a plaque in Old St. Paul's church." It strikes a responsive chord in many people searching for inner health. It goes, in part, as follows:

Go placidly amid the noise and the haste, and remember what peace there may be in silence.

As far as possible, without surrender, be on good terms with all persons. Speak your truth quietly and clearly; and listen to others, even to the dull and ignorant; they too have their story.

Avoid loud and aggressive persons; they are vexations to the spirit. . . .

Keep interested in your own career, however humble; it is a real possession in the changing fortunes of time. . . .

Be yourself. Especially do not feign affection. Neither be cynical about love; for in the face of all aridity and disenchantment, it is as perennial as the grass.

Take kindly the counsel of the years, gracefully surrendering the things of youth.

Nurture strength of spirit to shield you in sudden misfortune. But do not distress yourself with dark imaginings. Many fears are born of fatigue and loneliness.

Volunteering

Orville Kelly was, I think, a hero. Like anyone else, he was shocked and despairing when diagnosed with a deadly cancer. However, rather than give up and die, Kelly founded an organization called Make Today Count. This organization, with branches around the United States, encourages mutual support among people with life-threatening illnesses. It also served as one of the catalysts for the formation of many similar volunteer organizations.

Volunteer groups are, of course, helpful in providing information and resources to people in need. To my mind, however, the greater effect of these organizations is on the volunteers themselves. The act of helping similarly distressed or afflicted others is probably the most effective means of developing one's own network of healing social support. In addition to the close relationships that emerge, such volunteering provides purpose, commitment, and meaning to one's activities. Volunteer groups are most likely to benefit cholerics. Almost by necessity, cynicism, mistrust, and haughtiness give way when one is involved in helping others in need.

Kelly died of his cancer, lymphocytic lymphoma, after a seven-year battle. He lived much longer than expected. Kelly died just after winning a fight for veterans' disability benefits; he had traced his illness to exposure to nuclear radiation while in the U.S. Army. The details of his case remind us that emotions themselves do not cause cancer; the radiation did that. But the close ties and good feelings involved in helping others can help mitigate the health onsequences of environmental poisoning.

Buddy System

Another specific step that people can take to increase their social ties is to select a "buddy" for dealing with challenges. This buddy is simply someone else facing similar hurdles, who has agreed to work to develop mutual support.

This technique is most often used in groups of people fighting addictions, such as smoking, overeating, or drug use. An example I have seen of this process working at its best involves the case of Linda and Darryl. Linda, who had just quit smoking, called her smoking buddy Darryl every time she felt the urge to light up. Darryl talked her out of it and provided reassurance, and in so doing, strengthened his own commitment to avoid cigarettes. He also increased his own self-esteem.

Phlegmatics, who repress their feelings, are least likely to have such a helpful friend, although they are most likely to need one. Therefore, they are most likely to benefit from joining an organization that simply assigns buddies. It helps if the buddies are compatible, but they do not have to be lifelong friends.

Marriage

Married people live longer and healthier lives than do single people. This fact has many implications, and I will not try to begin a discussion of marriage. However, I cannot resist making one point.

What makes a marriage last? To find out what makes for a healthy, long-lasting marriage, interviewers sometimes simply go and speak to couples who have been happily married for many years. The couples report their observations. But the couples generally do not really know why their marriage succeeded.

Marriage and divorce rates vary by community, religion, age, state, era, country, economic status, and just about any other demographic variable you can name. These are generally not things over which people have much control. In other words, people *think* they know why their marriage lasted or why it failed, but in fact they are often wrong. If marriage and divorce depended heavily on the qualities of the individual, then marriage and divorce rates would be similar across time, places, and cultures.

These observations provide a clue as to the ways to maximize the chances of a successful marriage. The simplest and yet most important guideline is to place oneself in a context in which most marriages are successful. For example, a marriage of Mormons in Salt Lake City is much more likely to endure than is a marriage of actors in Beverly Hills. Of course, most of us fall somewhere in between these two extremes, but the principle still applies. If most of our friends are getting divorced, then perhaps we had better find some new friends to add to our social circle.

In the absence of marriage or a similar close relationship, some kind of structured self-disclosure is usually valuable, especially for phleg-matics. Depending on the individual, this may be anything from a pen pal to a planned rap session or even a diary.

Cooperative Ventures

The astronomer Carl Sagan has often appeared in the news urging that the United States and the Soviet Union plan a joint trip to explore Mars. What Sagan well recognizes is a principle that has been borne out in many psychological studies: people working together in pursuit of a common worthy goal often develop good relations with each other.

For cholerics, who may find it difficult to make friends and refrain from domination, cooperative ventures are often the key to self-healing. Once one begins working with others in a situation in which either everyone benefits or everyone fails, the aggressive, tense feelings begin to disappear faster than can be believed. Here again, the com-monsense advice to cholerics to relax and "get in touch with your feelings" is poor advice; instead, the place of the individual in the social situation is central. Of course, the ultimate goal must be team success rather than self-aggrandizement. Corporate mergers do not qualify as healthy cooperative ventures.

Some of the best cooperative ventures involve (amateur) team sports. Sports teams generally have a common goal, a feeling of camaraderie, a regular schedule, and the inherent interest of the players. As an added bonus, sports teams often provide a means of coping that goes well beyond the effects of social support—namely, the coping effects of exercise.

BIOLOGICAL COPING: CHANGING BODILY RESPONSES

Biological coping is probably the most misused and misunderstood aspect of the healing personality. Simply put, biological coping consists of those behaviors that directly modify the physiological components of emotional states. It is difficult to feel apathetic if you are in the middle of an auto race, and it is difficult to feel tense when you are being given a body massage on a warm Caribbean beach. In biological coping, we can move to directly eliminate our negative feelings, while ignoring their causes.

My evaluation of the evidence on biological coping differs from the conventional wisdom. I do not think that all of the techniques are for everyone. For example, some people simply should not meditate. And I do not believe that a fanatical desire to get in shape (physically or mentally) is very healthy. To explain the evidence for these views, I have divided the means of biological coping into three categories: exercise, systematic relaxation, and physical manipulation.

Exercise

There is no need to become a jogger. Jogging is a fine form of exercise for those who enjoy it, but a lot of people hate it. People should not feel that they have to become joggers, just as they do not feel that they have to follow a fad and become streakers. Each individual has to find the appropriate exercise. As I like to say, "Don't get exercised about exercise."

Exercise is an excellent means of biological coping because it almost always helps the body restore internal balance, especially if done properly. During moderate exercise, the body's metabolism is "tuned up"—blood is pumped efficiently throughout the body, the cells take in oxygen and sugar and excrete wastes, and the body's elimination systems go to work. And almost everyone can exercise. Exercise also can be used to improve psychological and social coping—going for a long walk with a friend can get you away from a stress-provoking job or home and provide an opportunity for venting feelings, while at the same time providing direct physiological benefits.

At age seventy-six, Katharine Hepburn reported rising at dawn every morning and swimming or bicycling or walking vigorously. This is an excellent example of good biological coping; these activities fall into a natural rhythm, are enjoyable, and usually are not overdone. Rose Kennedy swam and walked daily, even at age ninety. On the extreme, at age seventy, Jack LaLanne—perhaps the first American fitness guru—jumped into a harbor and, with handcuffs on, towed a flotilla of seventy boats. Jack LaLanne's exercise may have been appropriate for him, since he had spent his whole life developing his extraordinary physical fitness. For most people, his exercise would be fatal.

The evidence concerning the health effects of exercise was ambiguous until the publication in the mid-1980s of a long-term study of hundreds of Harvard men. In this study, the men who engaged in regular exercise were less likely to suffer a heart attack and lived longer overall. This study also reported another statistic, which I rarely have seen repeated. It was found that too much exercise was unhealthy! Most people are unlikely to exercise too much (that is, use more than 3,500 kcal per week), but this finding again points out the importance of balance. Exercise can be stressful if it is not appropriate for the individual.

There is also a small but real risk of sudden death from vigorous physical exercise. Jim Fixx, the author of the 1977 book *The Complete Book of Running*, probably did more than anyone else to popularize jogging. When he dropped dead of a heart attack at age fifty-two while out running, many joggers were shocked. They tried to explain that Fixx probably would have died at an even younger age if he had not taken up running. Maybe so, but there are many other athletes who have died on the tennis courts and jogging trails. There is no good evidence that college athletes live longer than their more sedentary classmates. Hard exercise is stressful and should be adjusted to the abilities of the individual.

In a discussion of psychology and health, I explained to a well-known psychologist that jogging has risks and may not be the best exercise for everyone. He exclaimed, "Then why am I getting up and doing that darned running every morning?!" He did not like the exercise, and it probably was not doing him much good.

The Best Exercise

Which exercise is best? First, the best exercise is the one that can be done regularly. This depends on circumstances. Horseback riding is not for city dwellers. Unfortunately, vacation advertisers often encourage the wrong approach. Northerners are urged to go swimming in the Caribbean, while southerners are told about the wonders of skiing in the northern mountains. They swim or ski for two weeks; then the vacationers return home and abruptly halt their exercise.

Second, exercise should not make one feel tense or angry. This depends on the match between personality and circumstances. If you are a choleric personality and racquetball leaves you feeling frustrated and disappointed, something is not working quite right. A melancholic Californian named Sue, who found her long walks on the beach terribly depressing, did much better when she switched to a water polo club. At age eighty, George Burns reported going for a brisk walk every morning while going over his monologues and songs; this worked well for him.

Third, it is best if exercise uses large muscle groups that move in a regular pattern. Walking and jogging are fine, but other helpful activities often are overlooked. For example, dancing, swimming, and cross-country skiing are generally safe, inexpensive, and relaxing.

These days, we hear a lot about "cardiovascular fitness through aerobic exercise." People are given formulas for computing their ideal pulse rate increases. They are instructed in exercise time, distance, and effort. You can see swimmers or bicyclists stopping to time their pulse. This is fine for a competitive sportsman or marathoner. But for the average person, it adds too much stress and confusion to activity that is supposed to reduce stress! This is yet another example of how the common wisdom about health leads one astray when a broader under-standing of the nature of good health is not achieved.

My simple rule of thumb is as follows. If I am exercising so vigor-ously that I cannot talk easily (without gasping and panting), then I probably am exercising too vigorously. On the other hand, if my body does not feel some stimulation or challenge (an "alive feeling"), then I probably am not exercising vigorously enough.

Interestingly, improvements in physical fitness have their greatest impact on health among those who are least fit. People who are moderately fit are much less likely to die than people who are unfit, but *super* fitness adds only a little more protection. A couch potato is likely to benefit from leaving the TV and going out for a daily walk, but a regular jogger is not likely to benefit from the addition of an hour of playing squash.

Exercise is especially good for melancholics. It is well established that vigorous activity can relieve depression. Depression involves inac-tivity, and it is impossible to be inactive when you are active. For similar reasons, exercise also is helpful for phlegmatics. Repressed inner tensions may be brought to the surface as the body's general level of activity is increased. For example, you might have heard a friend begin to disclose a series of personal problems after a vigorous game of tennis. It is very important for such people to institute a series of scheduled events—jogging partners, dance lessons, bicycle clubs—that will keep the exercise regular.

Exercise also is good for cholerics, but for a different set of reasons. The exercise allows cholerics to redirect their high energy and feelings of competition and aggression into the desire for high physical perfor-mance. As an added benefit, the muscle fatigue that follows exercise is incompatible with the tension cholerics usually feel. As a result, they relax. Aerobic exercise has been shown to reduce Type A behaviors while simultaneously improving general cardiovascular performance, even among the middle-aged. The tension of a marathon race is, however, probably less beneficial to cholerics than is the self-challenge of a long swim or a steep ski slope, although there is as yet no conclusive evidence on this point.

More than one marriage (and more than one life) has been saved when the couple instituted a program of daily brisk walks. For example, in one case the exercise encouraged the choleric partner to discharge his aggressive feelings and begin to relax. The exercise simultaneously encouraged the phlegmatic partner to feel enough motivation to begin talking about her repressed frustrations. The existence of the resulting discussion in an atmosphere removed from other distractions in turn led to realistic problem solving.

Reminder: Since too much exercise is a stress on the body, it is important for beginners to start very slowly and to receive a medical checkup. If your heart or circulation already is impaired, then a sudden and dramatic increase in physical activity can bring on a fatal heart attack.

Systematic Relaxation

Tighten both fists and hold them for ten seconds. Then relax your hands. Your hands will now feel especially relaxed. Contracting and relaxing our various muscle groups in a sequential fashion helps us to eliminate residual muscle tension of which we generally are unaware. Progressive muscle relaxation is a simple technique to promote general relaxation of the body.

In one recent controlled study, patients who were taught a simple relaxation technique lowered their blood pressure and LDL cholesterol in two months. In another study, of mostly older women in independent-living facilities, people were taught systematic relaxation and guided imagery in forty-five-minute sessions, three times a week for a month. Following the relaxation training, the people were found to have stronger immune systems (including enhanced NK cell activity) than did people in the control group, who did not receive the training.

It helps to focus on the part of the body in which one most often feels tension—for headache sufferers, the head, neck, and shoulders; for arthritis victims, the joints; for ulcer patients, the gut; and so on. (Yoga fans know of the idea of *chakra*, centers of energy in the body, waiting to be released.) For people with general anxiety, it is useful to start with the feet and slowly work upward. Regular practice is important—tense and relax, tense and relax.

Once the relaxation technique is mastered, it should be practiced in a relevant situation. For example, one man, an aggressive driver who became very angry in rush-hour traffic, gradually built up his muscle relaxation skills until he could deliberately go out in the worst of the rush hour and actively practice the relaxation. As with any conditioning, this practice involving a severe challenge helps the new reactions become easier and more automatic in less-challenging situations.

Systematic relaxation is a bad idea for many phlegmatics. They need to bring their inner conflicts to the surface, or at least to become more assertive and expressive. Practicing relaxation may simply encourage the ongoing repression of feelings. On the other hand, there is good evidence that relaxation training can alter the hostility of a Type A choleric.

Meditation (and Naps?), Etc.

In Xanadu did Kublai Khan a stately pleasure dome decree, but most individuals can conjure up their own Xanadus. Although it took an Eastern guru to bring meditation to the consciousness of the Western world, the meditative state is not really foreign to Westerners. Reveries, hypnotic suggestion, and quiet contemplation have a long history in Western literature and thought.

The essence of meditation is concentration. The feeling and state is one most people have experienced when totally absorbed in a good book, enthralled by a starry night, or hypnotized by a pounding surf. In such situations, we are peaceful and aware rather than tense and distracted.

Unfortunately, many habitations provide pounding headaches rather than a pounding surf. Or smoggy days without starry nights. And so we have to create our own individual state of absorption.

How do we know on what to concentrate? Some people, the more scientific and objective, simply concentrate on their own breathing. To do this, sit quietly in an isolated location and be sure that your body is relaxed (loosened clothing, comfortable seat, and so on). Listen to and feel your breathing. Your thoughts will wander, but bring them back to your breathing. Concentrate. Think of your body's cells being cleansed and rejuvenated.

For individuals positively predisposed to exotic Eastern religions, reciting a mantra like "wan wee wan" may be more effective than a focus on breathing. For those worried about heresy and wanting the Western, nonreligious mantra alternative, it is good to try repeating the number "one, one, one." Ambitious competitors can try focusing on saying "won, we won." (It doesn't hurt to add a little subtle humor to your meditation.)

If one wants to become more committed, there are a number of expensive and exotic-sounding books and courses that teach meditation. You can even get a personally assigned mantra. Unless one intends to become a guru, such books are not necessary for meditation, but they may very well build commitment to following up on one's investment.

Meditation really works for many people. That is, it decreases the stress-induced arousal of the sympathetic nervous system. Hence, it probably will be most effective for those who feel a lot of tension, hostility, or frustration. However, if you worry about whether you are meditating correctly, you should stop the meditating—or risk facing the severe stress of the Woody Allen character who forgot his mantra!

Let me now present a heretical thought that may cause some gurus to fall out of their mantras. For many people, naps work just as well as meditation. As the millions of inhabitants of many Latin countries understand, the early afternoon is time for siesta, the midday rest.

We cannot always find a place to take a nap. But many people can indeed go home for a lunch break, stretch out at a health club, or even find a couch in a private office. Physiologically, a midday nap makes good sense, since most workers experience a rapid drop in their blood sugar levels at this time, especially after a large midday meal. But not everyone feels this way. Some people have this low period later in the day, and it is silly to force them to rest at midday.

How does an individual know if a nap is healthy? You could probably find a medical clinic that would check your brain waves and your breathing patterns. An easier solution is this: Lie down and close your eyes after a calm, postprandial walk. If you cannot fall asleep, a nap is not for you. If you fall asleep but cannot wake up for hours, then you, too, must look elsewhere for relaxation. However, if you can fall asleep quickly and wake up about twenty minutes later feeling refreshed, then you have taken a step toward a healing personality. Why am I offering such seemingly obvious advice? Many people have never thought to try napping, or they think it is childish to nap.

Many religions prescribe prayer several times a day. This is not a bad recommendation as far as health is concerned. Prayer shares many elements with meditation. There is concentration, there is repetition, there is a peaceful self-awareness. A prayer break also disrupts any ongoing cycles of anxiety-producing thoughts. Less sophisticated but similar in effect are self-help groups that recommend taking a short break every morning, afternoon, and evening, repeating: "Every day, I try to be better in every way."

We do not know enough about the biological effects of music, but there is ample anecdotal evidence that at least some music can be inspiring, relaxing, and encouraging of inner balance. The famous conductor Bruno Walter (who lived to age eighty-six) wrote that music sends an "unchanging message of comfort: its dissonances strive toward consonance—they must be resolved; every musical piece ends in consonance. Thus music as an element has an optimistic quality."

Arriving in New York as a refugee in 1939, Walter was by no means a naive optimist. Yet music helped him transcend the horror of Nazi Europe and live in peace with himself. He wrote, "In spite of many painful experiences and the horror caused me by world happenings, I have always in moments of tranquility been conscious of a feeling of harmony."

Biofeedback

Despite its fancy name, biofeedback is, very simply, a form of systematic relaxation. What it adds is some equipment that helps us know when our bodies are tense. Although it is sometimes made to sound mystical, biofeedback is based on a simple principle: it is easier to maintain a relaxed state when we have information about the amount of stress we are experiencing.

We usually do not know how fast our heart is beating, how high our blood pressure is soaring, and so on. Biofeedback machines measure such internal states and give us this information. Some people, then, can learn to affect these internal states and thus reduce stress. There is no doubt that biofeedback works for some people, but there is also no good research showing that it is better than other forms of systematic relaxation.

Biofeedback is not for everyone. One middle-aged nurse with melancholic tendencies knew she could control her arthritis with vigorous daily swimming and eight hours of sleep every night. She needed activation, stimulation, and release. She did not need to be cooped up indoors with a machine that reminded her of her body's frailties.

Who should try biofeedback? There is no clear scientific evidence with which to answer this question, but my guess is as follows. Biofeedback is most likely to be helpful to people who have a lot of confidence in medical equipment and devices; who suffer intractable muscle-tension headaches; who have trouble recognizing when their body is distressed or relaxed; and in general, who are choleric, or possibly phlegmatic, but not melancholic.

Physical Manipulation

In many interviews I have read about Bob Hope, he talked about the benefits of massage. Even in his travels, he was either accompanied by a masseur or had a list of masseurs at his destinations. Physical manipulation in general, and massages in particular, are often an effective form of biological coping. Although these techniques have generally not been rigorously evaluated as to their effects on health, they are more than worthy of some reasoned speculation.

The benefits of massage come in several ways. The first is from the forced relaxation of tense muscles. As with systematic relaxation, meditation, and some forms of exercise, the relaxing of muscles leads to the easing of psychological tension. Healthy physiological responses then follow.

Massage and simple touching also seem to have direct psychophysiological effects. There is ample evidence that firm but gentle touching can be comforting. Most basically, children or other young primates who are raised without sufficient touching develop all sorts of distress and maladjustment. Problems ranging from skin rashes to adult sexual dysfunction have been traced to deprivations in touching at a young age.

A dramatic example of the use of touch to promote healing concerns the "King's touch" or "Royal touch" which was used by European kings throughout the Middle Ages as a supposed cure for scrofula (tuberculosis of the lymph gland). The technique of "laying on of the hands" is still quite popular among faith healers. Many self-help encounter groups also rely heavily on the perceived healing powers of touch. The beneficial effect seems to be based on humans' innate physiological need to be touched, intensified by the psychological powers often imputed to therapeutic touching.

Sex relieves tension. This is not my favorite bumper sticker, but it is true for many people. Because of society's general unwillingness to talk frankly about a basic biological urge, however, there is no good research investigating the effects of sexual relations on physical health. Undoubtedly, though, for some people the physical release helps restore a general homeostasis, whereas deprivation can lead to negative feelings. In addition, the emotional intimacy involved is healthy for the reasons already reviewed.

I do not know whether bakery workers live long lives. But it would not surprise me if they did. For many people, the smells of good food seem to have a relaxing, healing effect on the body. Some scientists have speculated that this is due to the very primitive and basic nature of our olfactory sense. My own best guess is that the benefits of good smells come mainly through pleasant associations. Smells have a remarkable ability to evoke memories of childhood that have long been forgotten—the smell of a campfire or a spring valley or a Thanksgiving dinner. The memories in turn often seem to create a state of relaxation and contentment.

Finally, as everyone should know, laughter reduces stress. It is physically impossible to be enjoying a deep belly laugh and to be nervous and uptight. In fact, one of the diagnostic criteria for an unhealthy Type A person is the lack of a belly laugh. Hearty laughter is different from having a sense of humor. A sense of humor can help us to think about stress in a better light; but uninhibited laughter seems to have direct physiological effects. A Ph.D. friend of mine does an excellent job of reducing tension with a glass of wine and the Three Stooges.

COMBINATIONS

Poor understanding of the three basic elements of coping—the thoughts, the social support, and the biological aspects—leads to some ludicrous theorizing about proper healing techniques. Someone may find that an Eastern religion or philosophy seems to promote inner balance and healing. Someone else may then "discover" that the key element for healing is yoga or meditation or concentration or dancing or chanting or whatever. Then someone else finds that meditation by itself is not as good as meditation combined with spiritual thinking. Then someone else adds praying. And so on. Prescriptions go around in circles until we are back to a new religion.

What is happening here, of course, is that self-proclaimed gurus are rediscovering that each element of coping can make a contribution to overall health. The same can occur in more traditional health care settings. One hospital may allow self-help techniques to develop, while another promotes prayer or meditation. One physician teaches visual imagery to her patients while another gives instruction in aerobic exercise. Each technique works some times for some patients but is not the whole answer. However, if the individual patient has a comprehensive understanding of where emotional imbalances come from and how they can be corrected, stable and meaningful health can be achieved, one that lasts a lifetime.

THESE DO NOT WORK

As a final thought regarding individual change, it is worth reviewing some commonly promoted self-help techniques that, as best as I can tell, simply do not work.

Subliminal suggestion tapes promise to relieve stress while you sleep, drive your car, or do your work. The bulk of the psychological evidence suggests that persuasive messages do not work unless you can consciously hear them. Once you can hear them, they are no longer subliminal suggestions.

Color therapy is sometimes advertised as a quick and simple means to adjust emotions. Although a cool blue room may be more soothing than a bright red room, the direct effects of colors are so minor as to be of no practical import on health. Of course, if colors are part of a totally redesigned work environment, then there may be measurable effects on stress levels.

Computer-synthesized music tapes or video images, hyped to "synchronize brain waves," are another far-out approach that seeks to capitalize on people's confusion about holistic healing. There is no computer-designed radio crystal that can tune one's brain waves.

Some fad diets, megavitamins, and other assorted potions also promise effects on emotional stability. It is, of course, true that psychoactive substances like caffeine, alcohol, and nicotine will affect one's physiology. It is true that certain foods are not tolerated well by some people. It also is true that gross disturbances in food intake (such as a big fatty meal just before bedtime) will affect physiological homeostasis. However, no diet that I know of (other than a reasonably balanced diet) has been shown to promote the emotional harmony of a self-healing personality.

We cannot eliminate challenge from our lives, and we should not try to escape it. Rather, to encourage healing emotions, we should measure and modify the match between our personal resources and the environmental demands. This can be accomplished gradually by changing both ourselves and our surroundings.

Once the best possible matches between the individual and the environment have been created, the focus of attention should shift toward coping with the remaining imbalances and stresses. With proper effort and practice, people can learn to alter their thoughts, their social relations, and their physical habits to combat the relevant distress.

Some of the needed changes cannot be done by ourselves. For example, a single individual cannot easily build a public dance hall, or create a volunteer organization, or change a hospital's patient care policy to allow greater personal control. The cooperation of many others is necessary. Society as a whole can either facilitate or thwart the development of self-healing personalities. The role of society is taken up in the next and concluding chapter.

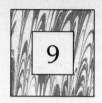

9

Is There a Health Conspiracy? What Can Society Do? What Will Future Research Bring?

Public opinion bubbles with conflicting stories about the role of personality in health and disease. Individuals struggle with uncertainty about the best ways to maintain their health. In reality, the facts are not at all confusing. The scientific evidence, when viewed *comprehensively*, gives clear reason to believe that the relationship between personality and health is real and important. It is not necessary to make outrageous claims. Simply put, there are disease-prone personalities, there are self-healing personalities, and there are things that can be done to change from the former to the latter. For many people, health and quality of life can be improved.

Chronic diseases, such as asthma, arthritis, cancer, migraines, ulcers, and heart disease, afflict hundreds of millions of people worldwide and cause untold suffering. To the extent that these maladies are promoted in part by psychological and social factors, immense opportunity exists for improving health. Careful examination and meta-analysis of assorted types of studies—of long-term epidemiological (population) research, of targeted studies of rats and lawyers and CEOs, of neuroendocrine studies of metabolism and immune function, of stress and illness in nonhuman primates, of social disintegration and social support, of the person-environment match, and of intervention studies to promote health—show that the evidence fits together in a consistent pattern.

Of course, not all distressed people succumb to illness and not all self-healing personalities achieve health. However, diet, smoking, blood pressure, amount of exercise, and other health risk factors are also imperfectly associated with health outcomes. My quantitative analyses of the size of the associations between emotional distress and disease repeatedly reveal that these links are of comparable magnitude to many of the more traditional health risks that people worry about. In fact, the risks to health from chronic hostility or depression are probably much greater than the risks of eating an egg a day or second-hand breathing a coworker's cigarette smoke.

In addition to the effects of stress-linked illness, millions more people suffer the health consequences of encountering emotionally distressed automobile drivers, apathetic safety workers, violent teen-agers, and so on. For still other people, stress stimulates smoking, drinking, overeating, and similar unhealthy behaviors. Although this book has focused on the direct internal links among psychosocial factors, emotions, and health, I also have noted the deadly effects of maladaptive behavior by the emotionally distraught. When these be-havioral links are added to the stress-mediated associations, the total effects of personality on health are astounding.

If I have made a sufficiently strong case in this book, then some will be inclined to respond, "Yes, well, that is reasonable and convincing; we will continue moving in the direction of promoting self-healing." But that would be a grave misperception. As I have demonstrated repeatedly, personality and stress factors are mostly *ignored* in health care.

The Heart Institute of the U.S. government's National Institutes of Health recently issued an important document—a list of cardiovascular risk factors to be used in conjunction with serum cholesterol levels in evaluating the threat of disease. The usual risk factors were there—family history, previous circulatory disease, smoking, diabetes, obesity, high blood pressure—but, incredibly, there was no mention of stress or hostility or any psychosocial variable! With a few notable exceptions, there is usually no reference to stress or emotions in advice to the public from cardiologists, oncologists, or other disease special-ists. And when stress is discussed, the meager advice offered may be years behind the existing knowledge. Importantly, no one has heretofore presented different recommendations for different personalities.

In the industrialized countries, about one-tenth of the gross national products are spent on medical care for people when they become ill. (That is 10 percent of all the money available for spending on anything, not just government spending.) Billions and billions of dollars more are lost in missed work. Is it unreasonable, then, to suggest that perhaps some of this money and these efforts would be better spent on developing individual interventions and psychosocial conditions that encourage and promote health?

IS THERE A HEALTH CONSPIRACY?

I often am asked whether there is a health conspiracy of doctors or drug companies or bureaucrats keeping patients away from simple and effective methods of self-healing. More and more people are becoming outraged at the dehumanization and coldness of much of health care, the inattention to family and community, and the emphasis on surgery and expensive drug treatments. They start to believe that there is planned manipulation—a health conspiracy to keep patients dependent on doctors.

People with arthritis wonder why some doctors cavalierly dismiss the diet, imagery, exercise, and health spa treatments they read about in popular health magazines. (In fact, many arthritis patients are helped by drug-free treatments.) Patients with chest pain question whether they really must go under the surgeon's knife. (In fact, too many coronary bypass operations are performed.) Patients with cancer are outraged if they are treated as a tumor rather than as a complex human being. Does the health care establishment conspire to keep patients away from self-healing treatments? No, there is not a conspiracy.

That is, government officials do not sit down with drug companies, physicians, and scientists, plotting to keep promising cancer treatments off the market. Physicians do not recommend surgery they know to be unnecessary. Scientists are not in cahoots with secret intelligence agencies to control the flow of new medical information.

However, the whole picture is not that simple. There is, in fact, an *unconscious conspiracy* of thoughts and medical traditions. New developments in understanding health often are indeed suppressed by a conspiracy of ignorance or an unplanned conspiracy of silence. For example, when there is a choice between a new drug treatment and a new exercise intervention, the health system will do a better job at instituting the drug regimen. For a patient with excessively high blood pressure or high blood cholesterol, it is easy for a physician to write a prescription for medicine (and almost criminal if the physician does not do something); but it is difficult for most physicians to prescribe and institute behavioral changes, such as stress-reduction training.

When there is a societal choice between psychosocial interventions and expensive, dangerous surgical interventions, the surgical interventions usually prevail. Few people question spending $20,000 or more of government money or insurance money on coronary bypass operations for workers with clogged arteries, but imagine the outcry if $10,000 were diverted from health funds to help a worker adapt to a stressful job!

When there is a choice between preventing illness and attempting to cure it, the health system will focus on the cure. The relative inattention to prenatal care as compared to newborn intensive care is a good (and scandalous) example. No hospital will let a premature infant die because the infant does not have health insurance, even if the newborn intensive care costs $200,000 (as it may). Many hospitals and obstetricians, however, will turn away a pregnant woman who cannot afford $1,000 for prenatal care that will reduce markedly the risks of an unhealthy, premature baby.

When there is a choice between conservative, homeostasis-oriented treatment and performing a costly surgery, the health system often errs on the side of intervention: excessive rates of tonsillectomies on children and hysterectomies on women are good examples from the 1950s and 1960s. (Current examples are, of course, hard to prove, but excessive cesarean sections are a likely case.)

It is very important not to blame individual health care practitioners for this state of affairs. Most health care providers work long hours under stressful circumstances. They deal with uncooperative patients, suffering, and death. They do what they think is best for their patients. Often they are very successful with their treatments. And they are happy to see patients recover, even if it is a so-called spontaneous remission.

There is no contradiction here between the establishment's failings and the practitioner's good intentions. Let me give an example from a different realm. In the early 1970s, when expectations about the roles of women and men were fast changing, I watched an excellent marriage of two fine people deteriorate. The wife was becoming more and more liberated. She went back to school, cut down on her housework, and asked for more equal treatment. Her husband tried but could not easily change. He had firm expectations for marriage from his own father, from his culture, and from the habits of their marriage thus far. He did not know how to cook or sew, but the big problem was that he did not know how to *think* about a different kind of marriage. The marriage failed, but neither partner was to blame.

In the same way, health care practitioners respond to the expectations of the system in which they work. Due to pressures from training, from peers, and from the medical environment, the individual practitioner has relatively little control over the medical tests and procedures that are expected to be performed, the treatments and referrals available, and even the fees and costs. Like marriage, the existing health care system is a traditional institution that does not adapt easily to changing demands. Successful changes in health care generally come from the top down—when the health structure and system change, individual practitioners follow suit.

RESISTANCE TO CHANGE

In the nineteenth century, physicians, nurses, and surgeons began the regular washing of their hands. They began to worry about the cleanliness of their instruments. They began to believe that perhaps it was they who were spreading infection in their own hospitals.

The idea slowly began taking hold that perchance there were germs that caused disease. Of course, most doctors thought this was ridiculous—imagine that tiny organisms that no one could see might be a cause of disease! Puerperal fever (caused by strep bacteria) was continuously being spread by doctors, nurses, and midwives to women in labor. Untold thousands of healthy young women died. Everyone "knew" (incorrectly) that the fever was caused by miasmas (poisonous vapors) or humoral imbalances or overly tight clothing on a swollen abdomen. The change to antiseptic operating rooms and gloved gynecologists took many decades.

Ironically, the idea of infectious agents like strep bacteria threatening health is so well established now that it has overwhelmed many other considerations in health. There are even people who suffer neuroses involving the excessive fear of germs. But the point is that we should not expect an immediate embracing of new approaches to healing.

Two centuries ago, infection was seen as an essential element of the healing process, since almost all wounds were infected. Infection characterized all who recovered from their wounds (not to mention all who died). Today, almost all patients are anxious and distressed, as an impersonal, isolating, disease-focused atmosphere is seen as requisite for proper medical care. Often I am told, "Of course patients are anxious, depressed, and angry; it is upsetting to become ill." Practitioners cannot "see" the unnecessary pressures that disrupt emotional balance.

Around the year 1870, Lord Lister of Edinburgh was able to establish standards of cleanliness and disinfection in surgery. The improvement in health was dramatic. Yet even at that late date, he faced ridicule and attack from unbelieving colleagues. Today, although improper handwashing practices remain a problem in many hospitals, "Listerism" has triumphed. But where will we find the Lord Lister of emotions and personality, the health leader who will change our approach to self-healing?

INTERVENTIONS

Dr. Walter Cannon began his 1930s book *The Wisdom of the Body* with a discussion of homeostasis in the body's organs and cells; but he concluded it with a discussion of social homeostasis. He was unwilling to write a book describing internal homeostasis and then ignore the obvious influences of an unstable social environment. With a reduction in social instability, Cannon wrote, healthy people would be freer to use their higher cortical functions to enjoy beauty, to explore the wonders of the world, to work, and to play. He thus presaged ideas of the self-healing personality.

What kinds of interventions can be and are currently being attempted to promote self-healing personalities? One important example of a possible societal action involves a research effort to help heart attack victims. In that study, over eight hundred victims of a myocardial infarction were randomly assigned either to receive or not to receive psychological counseling to reduce Type A characteristics. Over a period of several years, those receiving the counseling had a significantly reduced rate of recurrence of nonfatal heart attacks.

It is enlightening to examine the nature of the psychological intervention used in that study. It consisted of extensive instruction in progressive muscle relaxation, modification of exaggerated emotional reactions, self-management, ego strengthening, and establishment of new values and goals. Although such activities were aimed at reducing Type A behavior, it seems likely that such counseling also was effective in dealing with general anxiety, hostility, and depression, in addition to Type A behavior. Type A people were not being cured of Type A behavior, they simply were being trained to develop aspects of the self-healing personality.

Although this intervention study yields valuable proof concerning the role of personality in causing heart attacks, the evidence I present throughout this book suggests that it would have been much better if other aspects of personality also were measured, and if other diseases also were included. There should be less attention given to specific diseases and far more attention given to general disruptions in homeostasis. That is, the spotlight should be focused not on changing the Type A style of heart attack victims but on ways of promoting psychological well-being in the broader population. Such efforts will need to consider both the individual's personality and the environmental demands on that individual.

Another limitation of a focus on counseling heart attack victims is that it cannot be generalized easily to society at large. Should we give psychological counseling to the millions and millions of people who are theoretically at risk for cardiovascular disease (not to mention other chronic illness)? Even if we could afford such efforts, there are nowhere nearly enough trained psychological counselors. Such a Type A intervention approach follows the traditional medical model—

bring in some doctors to treat the Type A "illness"—and it is too narrowly conceived. Instead, a broader social view is needed. People need to change their own emotional reaction patterns and their social environments in ways that promote their health.

Can such society-wide changes be implemented? Generally speaking, an excellent example of a broad, successful change concerns cigarette smoking in the United States. Cigarette smoking has declined slowly but surely during the past three decades. The cumulative effects are dramatic, but the early going was rough. Evidence for the detrimental effects of smoking was "controversial," and most physicians smoked. It took a combination of factors to produce change. Some people have been helped to quit smoking by direct intervention—group therapy and individual psychological counseling—but that method solved only part of the problem.

The major influences on changed smoking patterns came from various changed social expectations. A number of factors contributed. The U.S. surgeon general issued increasingly stronger reports about the health risks of smoking. These reports were well publicized by the mass media. Physicians urged their patients to quit. Restaurants set aside no-smoking sections. Governments and businesses began to restrict smoking to designated areas, with some eventually banning indoor smoking altogether. Radio and television ads for cigarettes were prohibited. Tax rates on tobacco were raised. Antismoking advertisements were developed to compete with tobacco ads. Groups of activist nonsmokers began to form.

Each of these efforts had demonstrable effects, and together they were very successful. Importantly, each change affected certain types of people. Slowly but steadily, smoking came to be seen as an undesirable activity, even though most smokers do not develop cancer. In fact, with an intensive targeting on teenage smoking (when most smokers get addicted), the cigarette problem could be mostly eliminated in the United States within a decade. Similar large-scale efforts could be developed to promote a self-healing personality.

Successes

The last chapter looked at successful self-healing interventions for the individual. There are also many successful interventions in our communities.

On-site Crisis Counseling

Many police departments now have psychologists and other counselors available to help their officers through unusually difficult times. After a police shooting or a particularly gory accident scene, the police officer has somewhere to turn to deal with the feelings and begin to restore emotional balance. Police burnout (phlegmatic apathy) becomes less likely.

Many rape victims have described their interrogation by authorities and medical personnel as a second rape. The ignoring or disparaging of the emotional impact of being overpowered and raped led to ongoing distress. Today, many communities and hospitals have rape counselors available. Even better, a visit by such a crisis intervention counselor is sometimes mandatory. Help with the immediate emotional disturbances of being raped can prevent a costly physical illness from ensuing. Yet such counseling programs commonly find themselves struggling for funding.

Other crisis interventions that have proved successful are those for abused spouses, relatives of airline crash victims, and survivors of natural disasters. A generation ago such services were almost unknown. The presence of such interventions is one of the signs that a radical shift in the understanding of health is starting to take place.

Work-site Health Promotion

Johnson and Johnson, the large health care products company, has one of the best-established work-site health promotion programs. The "Live for Life" program is multipronged and includes a variety of exercise, relaxation, nutrition, and stress-management techniques. By having the program available in the workplace, employees do not have to travel to the program or worry about whether the interventions are legitimate. Plus there is the positive social influence of seeing co-workers taking part; yet each individual can choose what is most appropriate for his or her personality.

The Live for Life program also considers changes in the work environment. There are, of course, limits in the extent to which a job's requirements can be changed, but often the changes are not as disruptive as top management initially fears. For example, a worker may request an earlier lunchtime, a desk partition, a jogging path around the company's grounds, or a brighter color for the coffee room. The number of major American corporations with "wellness" programs has more than tripled during the past decade, another indication of the impending shift in how we think about health. Successful programs have been run by Xerox, Kimberly-Clark, and other huge businesses. Such corporate efforts are very valuable because they not only provide specific instruction and real facilities, but they also provide the powerful expectations that taking active steps to maintain health is a worthy goal.

Most professional sports teams now employ a sports psychologist or similar mental health expert. Although available for crisis counseling, the primary role of these individuals is to promote team morale. The best coaches understand that peak athletic performance depends heavily on psychological readiness—being "psyched." Performance falters when a player is in a "slump" (depressed), is "frustrated and jittery" (hostile), or is "tense and distracted" (repressed). It has always struck me as odd that sports fans would readily accept the idea of mental preparation for the challenge of a sporting event but would ignore the concept of mental preparation for the challenges of daily life.

Voluntary Peer Groups

A remarkable social movement that is on an accelerating trend in the United States is the growth of voluntary self-help peer groups. Women with mastectomies help new patients, reformed drug addicts help current addicts, overeaters help overeaters. As we have seen, these groups are especially valuable to individuals who are facing a chronic illness, since helping others is one of the best ways to improve their own coping skills. In general, many voluntary self-help peer groups are quite helpful in promoting a self-healing personality.

Examples of such groups include Reach to Recovery (breast cancer), the American Heart Association, Weight Watchers, Make Today Count (life-threatening illness), Alcoholics Anonymous and other "anonymous" groups, and the Phoenix Society (burn victims). Many other groups are local, with no national affiliations; referrals are made by local hospitals or town governments. Often, just the opportunity for an individual to see that others share the same problems is a tremendous help in restoring one's sense of emotional balance.

It is important that an individual not be forced to participate in such a group. If a person attends a few sessions and knows that participation is not helpful, then some other avenue should be sought that is more in line with that individual's personality.

Exercise and Recreation Facilities

It makes no sense to advise couples to take daily brisk walks in the park if the park is full of muggers or if there is no park at all. It is obvious when stated that there must be certain recreational facilities available for certain stress-reduction activities to take place. A conclusion of this book, however, is that such facilities must be available not only for the public's enjoyment but also for its *health*. Thus, it makes logical sense to think about whether public funds should be diverted from hospital construction to park maintenance. Although the thought is initially shocking to many, it reveals traditional biases and myopias concerning the nature of health.

Leadership

When President John Kennedy, a generation ago, announced a new effort to promote physical fitness, there was a tremendous response. School programs were reinvigorated and the sight of groups of people taking fifty-mile hikes became common. More recently, efforts by the

Reverend Jesse Jackson and other leaders have been attempting to show young people that they can take control of their lives and be healthy, fit, and accomplished. Such leadership efforts cannot work in isolation, but they are successful societal interventions that should be part of any ongoing efforts to improve health.

Interestingly, such calls to physical fitness are commonly accompanied by exhortations to public service, to caring for one's neighbor, and to living together in peace. I do not think it is an accident that leaders concerned with physical fitness also are interested in emotional harmony. They intuitively grasp what has now become scientific fact—that emotional harmony is part of true physical health.

Reformed Child Care

An early theorist in psychosomatic medicine traced most psychosomatic illness to the "infantile personality," which is basically an emotional immaturity carried into adulthood. The early work was based on clinical insights, mostly derived from psychoanalytic thought. For example, asthma was thought to be a result of childhood separation anxieties and excessive dependence on the mother. Although most modern researchers would quarrel with the idea of blaming adult illness solely on such notions as childhood separation anxieties, there is little doubt that many aspects of healing and disease-prone personalities have their roots in the child's development of a self-image.

There are libraries full of volumes explaining why children who grow up in predictable, loving environments and who develop a high sense of self-worth and personal competence are more likely to live healthier and more productive lives. Although no one knows how to raise the perfect child, there are many, many things we do know. Efforts to improve the social and emotional environments of children will pay off in terms of healthier adults. There is not yet enough data to estimate just how beneficial a stable, loving childhood will be, but it appears that it is the greatest single contributor to emotional balance.

CONTROLLING OUTRAGEOUS HEALTH CARE COSTS

In 1989, food inspectors in Philadelphia (who had been tipped off) found cyanide in two grapes that had been imported from Chile. In the panic that ensued, millions of dollars of fruit was destroyed. No further cyanide was found. Obviously, no one wanted to suffer instant death by cyanide poisoning. But people quite often suffer death from heart attack, stroke, and many other diseases from want of far less money than was lost on suspect fruit.

In the United States, the society generally has been unwilling to consider fully the costs versus the benefits of health care. Health care has been considered an individual's right, seemingly without limit. In fact, though, the limits are hidden. This illogical approach has led to bizarre situations in which Americans will selflessly donate thousands of dollars for hospital care for a dying child but will oppose a tax increase that will provide preventive health care to poor children or alter the health-damaging aspects of the child's environment.

This issue is especially relevant to the self-healing personality, because self-healing works over a period of time and in a social context. It cannot be administered in a two-week hospital stay. As general issues of health promotion and disease prevention become better understood by society, issues of emotional balance also may begin to receive the attention they deserve.

As noted, major businesses facing huge expenditures for the health care of their employees have turned increasingly to prevention, including techniques for stress management. Perhaps these experiences will provide a core of relevant data for instituting wider social changes. Unfortunately, the same nemesis returns here once again—the outdated, traditional medical approach to thinking about health. Because the psychological and social influences on health are not a major part of medical training, many physicians involved with company health plans are not fully equipped to implement and evaluate the psychosocial issues. So consultants are called in. But often the consultants, too, are insufficiently trained to do the job.

To compound the issue, there are also unfortunate economic structures in place regarding the healing personality. There are economic incentives for food companies to produce healthier food, and there are economic incentives in place for pharmaceutical companies to develop exotic drugs. There are similar incentives for diagnostic equipment, artificial organs, complicated new surgeries, and so on. But the economic incentives are mostly lacking for health approaches that seek to consider the individual and his or her role in the environment.

One simple but promising technique that has occasionally been tried is to make it pay to stay healthy. In some health insurance plans, patients who do not use much of their health insurance benefits for several years are given a monetary bonus or rebate. There is thus a direct economic incentive to stay healthy. The advantage to this approach is that it encourages people to think about those elements of health that are most relevant to them as individuals. The main limit of this approach is that there are bounds on how much people can do by themselves.

Cost Control

The new understanding of the self-healing personality has direct implications for cost control. There are four possible ways to deal with the current health cost crisis. The first is for workers and patients to pay more and more. They could pay either higher insurance premiums or higher taxes (or more in social security contributions). This increased spending route is the one that has been mostly followed in the United States, and the skyrocketing insurance premiums and budget distortions and deficits are the well-known result.

Second, physicians and hospitals could earn less. This could be accomplished through various sorts of laws that regulate the practice of medicine. Further direct government intrusion into the earnings of people in the health care industry does, of course, bring many problems of its own. Yet this is one path currently being followed. Canada and most European countries have a form of socialized medicine. In the United States, federal and state governments are capping the amounts they will pay for each Medicare and Medicaid patient for each medical condition. The administration of hospitals is being regulated.

Physicians' fees also could be controlled through programs that provide educational benefits, practice benefits, or other incentives to physicians in return for lower salaries. Many students would choose a medical career in public service if the right schooling and medical practice environments were offered to them. This type of approach is sometimes used in federal government hospitals but has largely been abandoned in the state and private sectors.

The third basic way to control costs is to degrade or ration the care. An outcry arose when the state of Oregon refused to fund certain organ transplants. Oregon is trying to pioneer a logical rationing approach to health funding. It has ranked health procedures according to their perceived public benefits, and it then funds the highest priority procedures until the funds run out. For some patients, there is no money for their risky, expensive operations, and they die. A sickly old man may be denied a liver transplant so that children can receive inoculations.

Most rationing, however, is hidden. Health is degraded as hospitals trim staffs and encourage the early discharge of patients. Physicians become less likely to recommend expensive procedures or order fancy tests that the patient cannot afford. Private hospitals "bump" and "dump" poor patients to public hospitals.

The fourth way to cut health care costs is *the only one in which there is no loser.* This solution simply involves keeping people healthier. In part it means promoting self-healing personalities. It means understanding individual needs and the individual's place in his or her world.

Because this solution to the health cost crisis is so clearly the best one, I am confident that it will be adopted eventually. The only question is whether it will be sooner or later.

NEW MEDICAL MIRACLES FROM THE MIND: DO THEY WORK?

New research studies of self-healing influences are published every day. New psychosocial and behavioral interventions are hawked in the marketplace. As new developments concerning health are reported, it is important to be able to evaluate them. Some are obvious shams, but others have a ring of truth. How should they be judged? There are two primary ways in which the individual consumer can decide if a newly announced development in this area is worthy of serious attention.

First, evaluate the new finding or treatment in terms of the material presented in this book. Does it make sense with respect to what we already know? Does it take into account individual personality, social demands, and chronic emotional reactions? I have reported dozens of important studies, including my own studies, that yield significant data about psychology and health. I have used hundreds of additional studies to develop the background material. If a new study contradicts the bulk of this evidence, we should be very suspicious of its validity.

Does the new research take into account and extend the existing evidence? Or does it simply examine a small, isolated piece of the puzzle? Unfortunately, many studies are not serious efforts by experienced investigators.

For example, every year or so there is a new study about the health effects (or lack of effects) of coffee drinking. Some claim that caffeinated coffee is bad, while others indict *de*caffeinated coffee. Some claim effects on cancer while others warn about heart disease. And so on. There is almost never any good theoretical reason to suspect a problem with drinking a couple of cups of coffee, and the findings never develop in a logical progression, one from the other. Compare these studies, on the other hand, to studies on the effects of marriage on health. As we have seen, there is excellent and varied theoretical reason to believe that married people lead healthier lives than do single people, and the findings of different studies are consistent on this point. My goal in writing this book is to present and clarify the main sets of findings concerning healthy psychosocial life-styles and to separate them from the trivial and contradictory bits and pieces of headlines that sometimes pass as health news.

The second way to evaluate new developments is in terms of the way the study was done. How many people were studied? Over what period of time? Who were they compared to? What measures were collected? How are discrepancies from past results explained? These are all questions that an intelligent layperson can and should ask. (And this information is reported by the better science reporters.) For example, if twenty women with breast cancer reported to their doctor that their cancer is getting better after they think about taking pleasant walks in the country, any conclusions should be regarded with extreme skepticism. On the other hand, a study that follows one thousand physicians for twenty-five years to see which psychological characteristics predict the development of heart disease should be taken very seriously.

The worst sort of evidence is testimonial. A very sincere-looking woman explains how her meditation (or diet, or faith, or exercise) regimen cured her cancer. Her healer stands nodding in the background. Although this sort of evidence is worthless, it is also the most common to be offered. We see it on television, in magazines, in books, and, of course, in "healing" meetings. In fact, such testimonials are so lacking in scientific merit that I use them as a sign of *lack* of efficacy; if any treatment is advertised with testimonials, my first presumption is that it is ineffective (or worse).

On the other hand, we cannot blithely assume that any conclusion from a government health agency or medical association is without bias. There are major ongoing turf battles in the health industry. Surgeons fight internists, psychiatrists fight psychologists, nurses fight doctors; and chiropractors, social workers, osteopaths, nurse-practitioners, and midwives all enter the fray. I do not think *fight* is the wrong word. The fighting is not physical, but rather involves bitter struggles in the legislatures, the courts, and the scientific journals. Each group self-righteously defends its own perspective, not to mention its own pocketbook.

On top of all this, we have the (often-legitimate) pressures and demands on research findings and interpretations exerted by the pharmaceutical industry, the food industry, the hospital industry, the medical supply industries, and the recreation industries, not to mention the antiestablishment populists. Each has a product that is seen to be more central and more important than all other influences on health.

The best quasi-governmental summary studies have been those that come from the National Academy of Sciences or its associated Institute of Medicine. The surgeon general's reports also have been mostly fair and accurate, although generally ignorant of the influences of personality and emotions. But overall, I believe the consumer can best stay on top of these controversies by sampling books in these areas and evaluating their plausibility in terms of our newly developed understanding of what it means to be healthy. The central issues and facts generally will become clear enough to the intelligent reader who delves beneath the headlines and takes new claims with a grain of salt.

MEDICINE OF THE FUTURE

In the next century, the popular understanding of health will change radically. We will discard the conception of disease as a bodily break-down that needs an overhaul in the medical repair shop. We will replace this outdated view with a more sophisticated outlook about health that is based on balance and homeostasis. Early signs of this impending change are there for the willing observer to see.

Today, if techniques to redress emotional imbalance are used in health care, they are employed as supplements to standard treatment. Is it not odd that the placing of foreign drugs and surgical scalpels into the body is seen as "standard," while the strengthening of the body's own healing systems is seen as ancillary and supplementary? Iron-ically, when this odd view is reversed, the drugs and the surgery work more effectively.

The final word is not yet in concerning the self-healing personality. Refined treatments for the phlegmatic, melancholic, and choleric pat-terns undoubtedly will be developed. I hope that increased public attention to the matters in this book will force the scientific community to accord them the serious consideration they deserve.

Although I have emphasized the broad scientific basis for understand-ing the self-healing personality, the personal rewards come from seeing individual results. As people learn to replace their negative emotions with healing ones, the resulting health is a joy that everyone can appreciate.

Notes

CHAPTER 1.
THE CHALLENGE OF HEALING

For an academic overview of the general field of health psychology, see my textbook: H. S. Friedman and M. R. DiMatteo, *Health Psychology* (Englewood Cliffs, N.J.: Prentice-Hall, 1989). For an advanced analysis of conceptual issues in studying the relations between personality and disease, see my edited volume: H. S. Friedman, *Personality and Disease* (New York: John Wiley & Sons, 1990).

For research on stress and diabetes, see B. Stabler et al., "Type A Behavior and Blood Glucose Control in Diabetic Children," *Psychosomatic Medicine* 49 (1987): 313–16. Also see V. Goetsch, "Stress and Blood Glucose in Diabetes Mellitus," *Annals of Behavioral Medicine* 11 (1989): 102–7.

Dr. Flanders Dunbar's book is *Mind and Body: Psychosomatic Medicine* (New York: Random House, 1955). The quote is from page 10.

For a description of healing at Lourdes, see R. Cranston, *The Miracle of Lourdes* (New York: McGraw-Hill, 1955); and P. Janet, *Psychological Healing* (New York: Macmillan, 1925). For a more general analysis, see J. D. Frank, *Persuasion and Healing* (Baltimore: Johns Hopkins University Press, 1961).

CHAPTER 2.
HOW CAN PERSONALITY BE RELATED TO HEALTH?

Cultural differences: see M. Zborowski, "Cultural Components in Responses to Pain," *Journal of Social Issues* 8 (1952): 16–30. A good description of national differences is given in Lynn Payer's *Medicine and Culture* (New

York: Henry Holt, 1988). For repetitive strain, see S. Kiesler and T. Finholt, "The Mystery of RSI," *American Psychologist* 43 (1988): 1004–15.

Twin studies: see, for example, T. J. Bouchard, "Twins Reared Together and Apart: What They Tell Us About Human Diversity," in *Individuality and Determinism*, ed. S. Fox (New York: Plenum, 1984).

The study of the Johns Hopkins students is described in B. Betz and C. Thomas, "Individual Temperament as a Predictor of Health or Premature Disease," *Johns Hopkins Medical Journal* 144 (1979): 81–89.

Many studies of biobehavioral mechanisms in heart disease are summarized in the July 1987 issue of the journal *Circulation*.

For a discussion of Type A and sudden death, see C. Brackett and L. Powell, "Psychosocial and Physiological Predictors of Sudden Cardiac Death After Healing of Acute Myocardial Infarction," *American Journal of Cardiology* 61 (1988): 979–83.

Hmong study: see J. Lemoine and C. Mougne, "Why Has Death Stalked the Refugees?" *Natural History* 93 (1983): 6–19.

A summary of Dr. Lown's work on arrhythmias is presented in B. Lown, "Sudden Cardiac Death," *Circulation* 76, supp. 1 (1987): I-186–96.

Dr. Saul's work is described in L. Saul, "On the Psychogenesis of Organic Symptoms," *Psychoanalytic Quarterly* 4 (1935): 476–83.

Stress of loneliness: see W. Stroebe and M. Stroebe, *Bereavement and Health* (Cambridge: Cambridge University Press, 1987).

Emotionality and stress: see C. Aldwin et al., "Does Emotionality Predict Stress?" *Journal of Personality and Social Psychology* 56 (1989): 618–24; S. Maddi, P. Bartone, and M. Puccetti, "Stressful Life Events Are Indeed a Factor in Physical Illness," *Journal of Personality and Social Psychology* 52 (1987): 833–43; and S. Stone and P. Costa, "Disease-prone Personality or Distress-prone Personality?" in *Personality and Disease*, ed. H. S. Friedman (New York: John Wiley & Sons, 1990).

CHAPTER 3.
STRESS: OUR CURRENT UNDERSTANDING

Walter Cannon: Cannon's classic book is *The Wisdom of the Body* (New York: W. W. Norton, 1932, 1939). His classic 1942 paper "Voodoo Death" was published in the *American Anthropologist* 44, 169–81. A good biography of Cannon is: S. Benison, A. Barger, and E. Walfe, *Walter B. Cannon: The Life and Times of a Young Scientist* (Cambridge, Mass.: Belknap Press, 1987).

Rat experiment: see C. P. Richter, "On the Phenomenon of Sudden Death in Animals and Man," *Psychosomatic Medicine* 19 (1957): 191–98.

Hans Selye: see his book *The Stress of Life* (New York: McGraw-Hill, 1956, 1975).

Life-change research: see, for example, R. Rahe and R. Arthur, "Life Change and Illness Studies," *Journal of Human Stress* 4 (1978): 3–15. See also J. Kaprio, M. Koshenvuo, and H. Rita, "Mortality After Bereavement," *American Journal of Public Health* 77 (1987): 283–87.

Rosetto study: see C. Stout et al., "Unusually Low Incidence of Death From Myocardial Infarction in an Italian-American Community in Pennsylvania," *Journal of the American Medical Association* 188 (1964): 845–49. See also J. Medalie and W. Goldbourt, "Angina Pectoris Among 10,000 Men," *American Journal of Medicine* 60 (1976): 910–21.

The stress of boredom: K. Orth-Gomer et al., "Type A Behaviour, Education, and Psychosocial Work Characteristics in Relation in Ischemic Heart Disease," *Journal of Psychosomatic Research* 30 (1986): 633–42.

Hamsters: see W. Tapp and B. Natelson "Consequences of Stress: A Multiplicative Function of Health Status," *FASEB Journal* 2 (1988): 2268–71.

Hassles: see, for example, M. Weinberger, S. Hines, and W. Tierney, "In Support of Hassles as a Measure of Stress," *Journal of Behavioral Medicine* 10 (1987): 19–31; and A. Stone et al., "Evidence That Secretary IgA Antibody Is Associated with Daily Mood," *Journal of Personality and Social Psychology* 52 (1987): 988–93.

Schwartz and Karasek: see R. Karasek et al., "Job Characteristics in Relation to the Prevalence of Myocardial Infarction," *American Journal of Public Health* 78 (1988): 910–18.

The Swedish sawmill study and similar studies of stress hormones were done by Marianne Frankenhaeuser; see, for example, "Sympathetic-Adrenomedullary Activity and the Psychosocial Environment," in *Research in Psychophysiology*, ed. P. Venables (New York: John Wiley & Sons, 1975).

CHAPTER 4.
NEGATIVE EMOTIONS AND HEALTH

For a discussion of hostility, see M. A. Chesney and R. Rosenman, eds., *Anger and Hostility in Cardiovascular and Behavioral Disorders* (Washington, D.C.: Hemisphere, 1985).

Disclosing traumatic events: see J. W. Pennebaker, J. Kiecolt-Glaser, and R. Glaser, "Disclosure of Traumas and Immune Function," *Journal of Consulting and Clinical Psychology* 56 (1988): 239–45.

The phlegmatic person: see H. C. Wood, *A Treatise on Therapeutics* (Philadelphia: J. B. Lippincott, 1976).

A good book on the psychobiological aspects of depression is Paul Willner's *Depression* (New York: John Wiley & Sons, 1985).

Bruno Bettelheim: see Bettelheim's *The Informed Heart* (New York: Free Press, 1960), 152.

Evidence for the role of depression in immune system changes is provided by S. J. Schleifer et al., "Major Depressive Disorder and Immunity: Role of Age, Sex, Severity, and Hospitalization," *Archives of General Psychiatry* 46(1) (January 1989): 81–87.

S. E. Keller et al., "Stress-induced Alterations of Immunity in Hypophysectomized Rats," *Proceedings of the National Academy of Sciences of the United States of America* 85(23) (December 1988): 9297–301. See also P. Gold, F. Goodwin, and G. Chrousos, "Clinical and Biochemical Manifestations of Depression," *New England Journal of Medicine* 319 (1988): 413–20.

Stress and voice tone: see F. Tolkmitt and K. Scherer, "Effect of Experimentally Induced Stress on Vocal Parameters," *Journal of Experimental Psychology: Human Perception and Performance* 12 (1986): 302–13.

For a general book on emotions, see C. Izard, *Human Emotions* (New York: Plenum, 1977). See also C. van Dyke, L. Temoshok, and L. Zegans, eds., *Emotions in Health and Illness* (San Diego: Grune & Stratton, 1984).

CHAPTER 5.
DISEASE-PRONE PERSONALITIES

Franz Alexander, *Psychosomatic Medicine* (New York: W. W. Norton, 1950).

The Yale study of breast cancer is: M. R. Jensen, "Psychobiological Factors Predicting the Course of Breast Cancer," *Journal of Personality* 55 (1987): 317–42.

Canadian study: see T. G. Hislop et al., "The Prognostic Significance of Psychosocial Factors in Women With Breast Cancer," *Journal of Chronic Disease* 40 (1987): 729–35.

Psychology and skin cancer: see L. Temoshok, "Biopsychosocial Studies on Cutaneous Malignant Melanoma," *Social Science and Medicine* 20 (1985): 833–40.

Depression, coping, and cancer: The early study of repressed, stoic response was S. Greer, T. Morris, and K. Pettingale, "Psychological Response to Breast Cancer: Effect on Outcome," *Lancet* 8116 (1979): 785–87; and K. W. Pettingale, "Coping and Cancer Prognosis," *Journal of Psychosomatic Research* 28 (1984): 363–64. See also P. J. Dattore, F. Shontz, and L. Coyne, "Premorbid Personality Differentiation of Cancer and Noncancer Groups," *Journal of Consulting and Clinical Psychology* 48 (1980): 388–94; D. Funch and J. Marshall, "The Role of Support in Relation to Recovery From Breast Surgery," *Social Science and Medicine* 16 (1983): 91–95; and D. Spiegel et al., "Effect of Psychosocial Treatment on Survival of Patients With Metastatic Breast Cancer," *Lancet* 8668 (1989): 888–91.

A description of Sandra Levy's work is in S. M. Levy, "Behavioral Risk Factors and Host Vulnerability," in *Psychological, Neuropsychiatric, and Substance Abuse Aspects of AIDS*, ed. T. Bridge (New York: Raven Press, 1988). See also S. Levy et al., "Survival Hazards Analysis in First Recurrent Breast Cancer Patients," *Psychosomatic Medicine* 50 (1988): 520–28; and S. Levy and L. Heiden, "Personality and Social Factors in Cancer Outcome," in *Personality and Disease*, ed. H. S. Friedman (New York: John Wiley & Sons, 1990).

The study of lung cancer mortality is: K. M. Stavraky et al., "The Effect of Psychosocial Factors on Lung Cancer Mortality at One Year," *Journal of Clinical Epidemiology* 41 (1988): 75–82.

Depression as a general risk factor for early death, Western Electric study: see V. Persky, J. Kempthorne-Rawson, and R. Shekelle, "Personality and Risk of Cancer," *Psychosomatic Medicine* 49 (1987): 435–49.

Johns Hopkins study: J. W. Shaffer et al., "Clustering of Personality Traits in Youth and the Subsequent Development of Cancer Among Physicians," *Journal of Behavioral Medicine* 10 (1987): 441–47.

An overview of Grossarth-Maticek's findings is provided in H. J. Eysenck, "Personality, Stress, and Cancer," *British Journal of Medical Psychology* 61 (1988): 57–75.

Cholesterol level and cancer: see A. Schatzkin et al., "Site-Specific Analysis of Total Serum Cholesterol and Incident Cancer in the HANES I Epidemiologic Follow-up Survey," *Cancer Research* 48 (1988): 452–58.

Studying Type A behavior: see S. Haynes and K. Matthews, "Review and Methodologic Critique of Recent Studies on Type A Behavior and Cardiovascular Disease," *Annals of Behavioral Medicine* 10 (1988): 47–59. See also T. Dembroski and P. Costa, "Coronary Prone Behavior: Components of the Type A Pattern and Hostility," *Journal of Personality* 55 (1987): 211–35; K. A. Matthews, D. C. Glass, R. H. Rosenman, and R. W. Bortner, "Competitive Drive, Pattern A, and Coronary Heart Disease: A Further Analysis of Some Data from the Western Collaborative Group Study," *Journal of Chronic Disease* 30 (1977): 489–98.

Norman Cousins: see, for example, Cousins's book *The Healing Heart* (New York: W. W. Norton, 1983).

Two of my own studies in the area of Type A behavior are: H. S. Friedman, J. Hall, and M. Harris, "Type A Behavior, Nonverbal Expressive Style, and Health," *Journal of Personality and Social Psychology* 48 (1985): 1299–1315; and H. S. Friedman and S. Booth-Kewley, "Personality, Type A Behavior and Coronary Heart Disease," *Journal of Personality and Social Psychology* 53 (1987): 783–92.

George Burns: see his *Living It Up* (New York: Putnam, 1976), 11.

Retirement: see A. Antonovsky, "Personality and Health: Testing the

Sense of Coherence Model," in *Personality and Disease*, ed. H. S. Friedman (New York: John Wiley & Sons, 1990). See also A. Leaf, "Getting Old," *Scientific American* 229 (1973): 44–52.

Pablo Casals quote: from H. L. Kirk, *Pablo Casals: A Biography* (New York: Holt, Rinehart, Winston, 1974), 504.

Social class and disease proneness: see G. Rose and M. Marmot, "Social Class and Coronary Heart Disease," *British Heart Journal* 45 (1981): 13–19. See also R. Karasek et al., "Job, Psychological Factors and Coronary Heart Disease," *Advances in Cardiology* 29 (1982): 62–67.

Type A and control: see, for example, D. Glass et al., "Effects of Harassment and Competition Upon Cardiovascular and Plasma Catecholamine Response in Type A and Type B Individuals," *Psychophysiology* 17 (1980): 453–63. M. E. P. Seligman, *Helplessness: On Depression, Development and Death* (San Francisco: Freeman, 1975).

Animal tumors: see B. Fox and B. Newberry, eds., *Psychoneuroendocrine Systems in Cancer and Immunity* (Toronto: Hogrefe, 1984). Also see K. Bammer and B. Newberry, eds., *Stress and Cancer* (Toronto: Hogrefe, 1981).

Worrying about worry: see A. Bandura, "Self-efficacy Conception of Anxiety," *Anxiety Research* 1 (1988): 77–98.

The study of Harvard men and pessimism is C. Peterson, M. E. P. Seligman, and G. E. Vaillant, "Pessimistic Explanatory Style Is a Risk Factor for Physical Illness," *Journal of Personality and Social Psychology* 55 (1988): 23–27.

Suspiciousness and cynicism: see J. C. Barefoot et al., "Suspiciousness, Health, and Mortality," *Psychosomatic Medicine* 49 (1987): 450–57; and A. Ostfeld et al., "A Prospective Study of the Relationship Between Personality and Coronary Heart Disease," *Journal of Chronic Disease* 17 (1964): 265–76.

The Tecumseh study is described in M. Julius et al., "Anger-Coping Types, Blood Pressure, and All-Cause Mortality," *American Journal of Epidemiology* 124 (1986): 220–33.

For a discussion of alexithymia, see I. Lesser, "A Review of the Alexithymia Concept," *Psychosomatic Medicine* 43 (1981): 531–43. See also O. Todarello et al., "Alexithymia and Breast Cancer," *Psychotherapy and Psychosomatics* 51 (1989): 51–55.

For discussions of emotional expressivity and disease, see R. Buck, *The Communication of Emotion* (New York: Guilford Press, 1984); and C. Malatesta, R. Jones, and C. Izard, "The Relation Between Low Facial Expressivity During Emotional Arousal and Somatic Symptoms," *British Journal of Medical Psychology* 60 (1987): 169–80. For a review regarding cancer, see J. Gross, "Emotional Expression in Cancer Onset and Progression," *Social Science and Medicine* 28 (1989): 1239–48.

My major published meta-analysis is: H. S. Friedman and S. Booth-Kewley, "The Disease-Prone Personality: A Meta-analytic View of the Construct," *American Psychologist* 42 (1987): 539–55. See also S. Booth-Kewley and H. S. Friedman, "Psychological Predictors of Heart Disease," *Psychological Bulletin* 101 (1987): 343–62.

Biology of arthritis: see E. M. Sternberg et al., "Inflammatory Mediator-Induced Hypothalamic-Pituitary-Adrenal Axis Activation Is Defective in Streptococcal Cell Wall Arthritis-Susceptible Lewis Rats," *Proceedings of the National Academy of Sciences* 86 (1989): 2374–78.

Immune system functioning and arthritis: see A. Zautra et al., "Life Stress and Lymphocyte Alterations Among Patients With Rheumatoid Arthritis," *Health Psychology* 8 (1989): 1–14. See also S. Levy et al., "Persistently Low Natural Killer Cell Activity in Normal Adults: Immunological, Hormonal, and Mood Correlates," *Natural Immune Cell Growth Regulation* 8 (1989): 173–86.

Arthritic personality myth: see P. Spergel, G. Ehrlich, and D. Glass, "The Rheumatoid Arthritic Personality: A Psychodiagnostic Myth," *Psychosomatics* 19 (1978): 79–86.

For a study of conditioned allergic response in rats, see G. MacQueen et al., "Pavlovian Conditioning of Rat Mucosal Mast Cells to Secrete Rat Mast Cell Protease II," *Science* 243 (1989): 83–85.

William Beaumont: *Experiments and Observations on the Gastric Juice and the Physiology of Digestion* (Plattsburgh, N.Y.: E. P. Allen, 1833).

Rats, men, and ulcers: see J. Weiss, "Effects of Coping Behavior in Different Warning Signal Conditions of Stress Pathology in Rats," *Journal of Comparative and Physiological Psychology* 77 (1971): 1–13; and P. Walker et al., "Life Events Stress and Psychosocial Factors in Men With Peptic Ulcer Disease," *Gastroenterology* 94 (1988): 323–30.

Women and ulcers: see C. B. Travis, *Women and Health Psychology* (Hillsdale, N.J.: Erlbaum, 1988).

Combined risk factors: see K. Perkins, "Interactions Among Coronary Heart Disease Risk Factors," *Annals of Behavioral Medicine* 11 (1989): 3–11.

Washington University study of depression and heart attack: R. Carney et al., "Major Depressive Disorder Predicts Cardiac Events in Patients With Coronary Artery Disease," *Psychosomatic Medicine* 50 (1988): 627–33.

Canadian study: J. Murphy et al., "Affective Disorders and Mortality," *Archives of General Psychiatry* 44 (1987): 473–80; see p. 479 for quoted material.

CHAPTER 6.
PERSONALITIES THAT RESIST DISEASE:
THE SELF-HEALING PERSONALITY

For a discussion of the idea of "health" versus "disease," see A. Antonovsky, *Health, Stress, and Coping* (San Francisco: Jossey Bass, 1979).

Children with strep: see R. Meyer and R. Haggerty, "Strepococcal Infections in Families," *Pediatrics* 29 (1962): 539–49.

Stress among executives and lawyers: see S. Maddi and S. Kobasa, *The Hardy Executive* (Chicago: Dorsey Press, 1984); J. Barefoot et al., "The Cook-Medley Hostility Scale: Item Content and Ability to Predict Survival," *Psychosomatic Medicine* 51 (1989): 46–57; and S. Kobasa, "Commitment and Coping in Stress Resistance Among Lawyers," *Journal of Personality and Social Psychology* 42 (1982): 707–17.

M. F. Scheier et al., "Dispositional Optimism and Recovery from Coronary Artery Bypass Surgery: The Beneficial Effects on Physical and Psychological Well-being," *Journal of Personality and Social Psychology* 57, 6 (1989): 1024–40.

Harvard Magazine column by John Train: January–February 1989, p. 6.

Workers' sense of control and health: see S. Cobb and S. Kasl, *Termination: The Consequences of Job Loss*, Report prepared for the U.S. Department of Health, Education, and Welfare (Washington, D.C.: Government Printing Office, 1977). See also J. Rodin, "Health, Control, and Aging," in *The Psychology of Control and Aging*, ed. M. Baltes and P. Baltes (Hillsdale, N.J.: Erlbaum, 1986).

Mary Decker Slaney's quote is from *American Health* (June 1989): 68. Arthur Schopenhauer's remark is in *Essays on Personality; or What a Man Is*.

For analyses of the physiological benefits of stress, see, for example, R. A. Dienstbier, "Arousal and Physiological Toughness," *Psychological Review* 96 (1989): 84–100; and R. A. Martin et al., "Is Stress Always Bad?" *Journal of Personality and Social Psychology* 53 (1987): 970–82. See also H. J. Eysenck and M. W. Eysenck, *Personality and Individual Differences* (New York: Plenum, 1985).

William James is quoted from *The Principles of Psychology* (New York: Henry Holt and Company, 1890), 97.

Abraham Maslow: see his *Motivation and Personality*, 2d ed. (New York: Harper & Row, 1970).

For studies of social integration and other relevant sociocultural factors, see S. L. Syme, "Coronary Artery Disease: A Sociocultural Perspective," *Circulation* 76 (1987): I-112–16; T. E. Seeman et al., "Social Network Ties and Mortality Among the Elderly in the Alameda County Study," *American Journal of Epidemiology* 126 (1987): 714–23; and G. E. Moss, *Illness, Immunity, and Social Interaction* (New York: John Wiley & Sons, 1973).

Aaron Antonovsky's case of the holocaust survivor is described in *Unraveling the Mystery of Health* (San Francisco: Jossey-Bass, 1987). See also Viktor Emil Frankl, *Man's Search for Meaning: An Introduction to Logotherapy. A newly revised and enlarged ed. of From Death-camp to Existentialism*. Trans. by Ilse Lasch, preface by Gordon W. Allport (New York: Simon & Schuster, 1962).

CHAPTER 7.
INNER HEALING THROUGH NERVES AND HORMONES

For good reports on nutrition and health, see U.S. Public Health Service, *The Surgeon General's Report on Nutrition and Health* (Washington, D.C.: Government Printing Office, 1988); and P. Saltman, J. Gurin, and I. Mothner, *The California Nutrition Book* (Boston: Little, Brown, 1987).

For cholesterol and cancer, see A. Schatzkin et al., "Site-Specific Analysis of Total Serum Cholesterol and Incident Cancer in NHANES I," *Cancer Research* 48 (1988): 452–58.

Some old but relevant studies showing the link between stress and cholesterol are S. Wolf et al., *Circulation* 26 (1962): 379–87; S. Grundy and A. Griffin, *Circulation* 17 (1958): 852; and C. B. Murphy et al., *Journal of Chronic Disease* 8 (1958): 661.

For a discussion of Type A personality and physiological reactivity, see T. J. Harbin, "The Relationship Between the Type A Behavior Pattern and Physiological Reactivity," *Psychophysiology* 26 (1989): 110–19.

For a discussion of stress and hormones, see M. Lader, "Anxiety and Depression," in *Physiological Correlates of Human Behavior*, vol. 3, ed. A. Gale and J. Edwards (London: Academic Press, 1983). See also J. Rodin, "Health, Control, and Aging," in *Psychology of Control and Aging*, ed. M. Baltes and P. Baltes (Hillsdale, N.J.: Erlbaum, 1986).

For discussions of stress and the immune system, see J. Jemmott and S. Locke, "Psychosocial Factors, Immunologic Mediation, and Human Susceptibility to Infectious Diseases," *Psychological Bulletin* 95 (1984): 78–108; and R. Glaser et al., "Stress-Related Immune Suppression," *Brain, Behavior, and Immunity* 1 (1987): 7–20.

For studies of stress and atherosclerosis in monkeys, see S. Manuck et al., "Effects of Stress and the Sympathetic Nervous System on Coronary Artery Atherosclerosis in the Cynomolgus Macaque," *American Heart Journal* 116 (1988): 328–33. For a paper on personality, physiological reactivity, diet, and heart disease, see N. Schneiderman, "Psychophysiologic Factors in Atherogenesis and Coronary Artery Disease," *Circulation* 76 (1987): 41–47.

For Dr. Robert Sapolsky's work, see R. M. Sapolsky, "The Endocrine Stress-Response and Social Status in the Wild Baboon," *Hormones and Behavior* 16 (1982): 279; R. M. Sapolsky, "Stress-Induced Elevation of Testosterone Concentrations in High Ranking Baboons: Role of Catecholamines," *Endocrinology* 118 (1986): 1630–35; and R. M. Sapolsky and G. Mott, "Social Subordinance in Wild Baboons Is Associated With Suppressed High Density Lipoprotein-Cholesterol Concentrations," *Endocrinology* 121 (1987): 1605–10. Sex hormones: see H. H. Feder, "Hormones and Sexual Behavior," *Annual Review of Psychology* 35 (1984): 165–200.

The study of New Zealand rabbits is C. Tsopanakis et al., "Effects of Cold

Stress on Serum Lipids, Lipoproteins, and the Activity of Lecithin: Cholesterol Acyltransferase in Rabbits," *Biochemical Medicine and Metabolic Biology* 39 (1988): 148–57.

Blue-collar workers and stress: see J. Siegrist et al., "Atherogenic Risk in Men Suffering From Occupational Stress," *Atherosclerosis* 69 (1988): 211–18. See also A. Baum, R. Fleming, and D. Reddy, "Unemployment Stress," *Social Science and Medicine* 22 (1986): 509–16.

For Type B reactivity, see M. Muranaka et al., "Stimulus-Specific Patterns of Cardiovascular Reactivity in Type A and B Subjects," *Psychophysiology* 25 (1988): 330–38.

Endorphins and cholesterol in mice: see H. Bryant et al., "Stress and Morphine-Induced Elevations of Plasma and Tissue Cholesterol in Mice," *Biochemical Pharmacology* 37 (1988): 3777–80.

The role of the hemispheres in emotional repression is discussed in R. Davidson, "Affect, Repression, and Cerebral Asymmetry," in *Emotions in Health and Illness*, ed. L. Temoshok, C. van Dyke, and L. Zegans (New York: Grune & Stratton, 1983).

For an overview of James Pennebaker's work, see J. W. Pennebaker, "Confession, Inhibition, and Disease," *Advances in Experimental Social Psychology* 22 (1989): 211–44. See also L. Jamner, G. Schwartz, and H. Leigh, "The Relationship Between Repressive and Defensive Coping Styles and Monocyte, Eosinophile, and Serum Glucose Levels," *Psychosomatic Medicine* 50 (1988): 567–75.

Stress, nervous system response, and immune system function: see J. Kiecolt-Glaser and R. Glaser, "Behavioral Influences on Immune Function," in *Stress and Coping Across Development*, ed. T. Field (Hillsdale, N.J.: Erlbaum, 1988); and J. M. Weiss et al., "Behavioral and Neural Influences on Cellular Immune Responses," *Journal of Clinical Psychiatry* 50, supp. (1989): 43–53.

CHAPTER 8.
ACHIEVING HOMEOSTASIS:
DEVELOPING A SELF-HEALING PERSONALITY

Benjamin Franklin, *Autobiography and Other Pieces*, edited with an introduction by Dennis Welland (London: Oxford University Press, 1970).

The U-shaped relation to serum cholesterol is described in H. Iso et al., "Serum Cholesterol Levels and Six-Year Mortality From Stroke," *New England Journal of Medicine* 320 (1989): 906.

The study of hospital roommates is: J. Kulik and H. Mahler, "Effects of Preoperative Roommate Assignment on Anxiety and Recovery From Coronary Bypass Surgery," *Health Psychology* 6 (1987): 525–43.

The work of Irving Janis is described in I. L. Janis, *Stress and Frustration* (New York: Harcourt Brace Jovanovich, 1969).

Kai Erikson's study of the flood is: K. Erikson, *Everything in Its Path: Destruction of Community in the Buffalo Creek Flood* (New York: Simon & Schuster, 1969). The quote is from p. 240.

For thinking about life tasks, see, for example, N. Cantor et al., "Life Tasks, Self-concept Ideals, and Cognitive Strategies in a Life Transition," *Journal of Personality and Social Psychology* 53 (1987): 1178–91.

The Salk quote is from *50 Plus* magazine (July 1985): 48.

The study of Japanese-Americans is: M. Marmot and L. Syme, "Acculturation and Coronary Heart Disease in Japanese-Americans," *American Journal of Epidemiology* 104 (1976): 225–46.

Social support strategies are described in more detail in B. H. Gottlieb, *Social Support Strategies* (Beverly Hills: Sage, 1983).

For studies of exercise and health, see Paffenberger et al., "A Natural History of Athleticism and Cardiovascular Health," *Journal of the American Medical Association* 252 (1984): 491–95 (the Harvard study). See also H. W. Kohl, R. LaPorte, and S. Blair, "Physical Activity and Cancer," *Sports Medicine* 6 (1988): 222–37; S. Blair et al., "Physical Fitness and All Cause Mortality," *Journal of the American Medical Association* 262 (1989): 2395–401; J. Blumenthal et al., "Exercise Training in Healthy Type A Middle-aged Men," *Psychosomatic Medicine* 50 (1988): 418–33; and C. Ross and D. Hayes, "Exercise and Psychologic Well-being in the Community," *American Journal of Epidemiology* 127 (1988): 762–71.

Relaxation technique and coronary risk: see M. Carson et al., "The Effect of a Relaxation Technique on Coronary Risk Factors," *Behavioral Medicine* 14 (1988): 71–77; and E. Nunes, K. Frank, and D. Kornfeld, "Psychologic Treatment for the Type A Behavior Pattern and for Coronary Heart Disease," *Psychosomatic Medicine* 48 (1987): 159–73. And immunity: see J. Kiecolt-Glaser et al., "Psychosocial Enhancement of Immunocompetence in a Geriatric Population," *Health Psychology* 4 (1985): 25–41.

Bruno Walter: see his *Theme and Variations: An Autobiography*, trans. J. A. Galston (New York: Knopf, 1946), 341.

Touching and health: see A. Montague, *Touching: The Human Significance of the Skin* (New York: Harper & Row, 1978).

CHAPTER 9.
IS THERE A HEALTH CONSPIRACY?
WHAT CAN SOCIETY DO?
WHAT WILL FUTURE RESEARCH BRING?

On the idea of a health conspiracy, see I. Illich, *Medical Nemesis: The Expropriation of Health* (New York: Pantheon, 1976). See also T. Szasz, *The Theology of Medicine* (Baton Rouge: Louisiana State Press, 1977).

For studies of Cesarean section, see: P. J. Placek and S. M. Taffel, "Vaginal

Birth after Cesarean (VBAC) in the 1980s," *American Journal of Public Health* 78(5) (1988): 512–15. S. M. Taffel, P. J. Placek, and T. Liss, "Trends in the United States Cesarean Section Rate and Reasons for the 1980–85 Rise," *American Journal of Public Health* 77 (8) (1987): 955–59.

The study of interventions to prevent recurrent heart attacks is M. Friedman et al., "Alteration of Type A Behavior and Its Effects on Cardiac Recurrences in Post Myocardial Infarction Patients," *American Heart Journal* 112 (1986): 653–65.

For a discussion of work-site health promotion, see K. Pelletier, *Healthy People in Unhealthy Places* (New York: Delta, 1984).

Disease prevention: see R. M. Kaplan and M. Criqui, eds., *Behavioral Epidemiology and Disease Prevention* (New York: Plenum, 1985).

The idea of the infantile personality: see J. Ruesch, "The Infantile Personality: The Core Problem of Psychosomatic Medicine," *Psychosomatic Medicine* 10 (1948): 134–44.

Index

Accidents, 152

Acquired immune deficiency syndrome (AIDS), 139, 149–50

Addictive personality, 25–26

Adrenal cortex, 136

Adrenal glands, 35, 135

Adrenaline, 135, 137, 140

Aerobic exercise, 192–93

Aesop's Fables, 46

Affective (mood) disorder, 93–94

Aggression. *See* Hostility and aggression

AIDS, 139, 149–50

Alameda County, California, study in, 124, 183

Alcoholics Anonymous, 212

Alexander, Dr. Franz, 57, 64

Allergens, 87

American Cancer Society, 132

American Heart Association, 132, 212

Anger, 46, 47, 50, 71, 75
dealing with creeps, 182
physical illness and, 87, 89
repression of. *See* Repression

Angina, 26–27

Antonovsky, Aaron, 126

Anxiety, 46–47, 72

chronic, 46
healthy, 46
physical illness and, 97
arthritis, 85
asthma, 87, 88
death, 93–94
headaches, 88, 89
ulcers, 90, 91

Anxiety disorder, 47

Apathy, 48–51, 75, 169
challenge and, 111
versus depression, 50, 51
immune system-related disease and, 139
phony Type B behavior, 71
repression and, 49–50, 80–81
survival of cancer and, 60. *See also* Self-healing personality

Apocrypha, 64

Arousal reduction, 112

Arteries, plaque buildup in, 23, 135, 137. *See also* Atherosclerosis

Arthritis, 1, 2, 23, 24, 84, 85–86, 204

Asthma, 1, 2, 84, 86–88, 151

Atherosclerosis, 137, 142, 162
high blood pressure and, 135
hostility and, 67, 140–41
monkey studies, 140–41

Baboons, studies with, 141–42
Back pain, low, 86
Bacon, Sir Francis, 17
B cells, 139
Beaumont, Dr. William, 89
Becker, Boris, 116
Becket, Thomas à, 8
Behavioral links between personality and health, 25–26, 97, 149, 152–53, 203
Bereavement, 139
Bernard, Dr. Claude, 33
Bettelheim, Bruno, 50
Biofeedback, 197–98
Biological coping, 167, 190–99
   biofeedback, 197–98
   exercise, 167, 190–94
   meditation, 157, 195–97
   physical manipulation, 198–99
   systematic relaxation, 167, 194–95
Blaming the victim, 94–96
Blood pressure, 64, 127–28, 135, 194
   high. *See* Hypertension
   mood and, 42
Booth-Kewley, Stephanie, 73, 82
Boredom, 111
Brain
   multiple, 145–146. *See also* Nervous system
Breast cancer, 160, 212
   personality and survival of, 57–58, 59, 60, 139
Buddy system, 188
Business associates, 185
Brynner, Yul, 110–11
Burns, George, 4, 72–73, 192

Caesar, Julius, 24
Cancer, 1, 2, 23–24, 62–63
   blaming the victim, 94, 95, 96
   cholesterol levels and, 62, 133, 137–38

fear of, 148
immune system and, 149
personality and development of, 60–63, 104, 149, 162
   helplessness, 77
   suspiciousness, 79
personality and survival of, 57–59, 60, 63, 104, 111, 139, 162
unproven drugs, 7, 8
Cannon, Dr. Walter, 30, 31, 32, 33, 53, 113, 207
Canterbury Tales, The (Chaucer), 7–8
Cardiac arrhythmias, 24
Cardiovascular diseases, 148. *See also specific forms of cardiovascular disease*
Carret, Philip, 105–6
Casals, Pablo, 4, 73, 119
Catecholamine-depleting drugs, 51
Catecholamines, 135, 137, 140, 148
Cerebellum, 146
Cerebrum, 146
Challenge, viewing life as a, 103, 104, 110–13, 127
   emotional training, 112
Change. *See* Life changes, major
Chaucer, Geoffrey, 7
Cheerfulness, 118
Chief executive officers (CEOs), 102
Childbirth, hospital environment during, 107–8
Child care, reformed, 213
Choleric people. *See* Hostility and aggression
Cholesterol, 62, 129–33, 137–38, 142, 143, 144, 150, 163, 194
Cholinergic agonists, 51
Cigarette smoking, societal efforts to eliminate, 209
Cirrhosis, 150
Coffee drinking, 217
Coherence, 126

Color therapy, 200–201
Commitment, sense of, health and, 102–3, 104–5, 109–10, 127
Community, social ties in the, 124
Competence, 106
Competitiveness, 64, 76
Computer-synthesized tapes to "synchronize brain waves," 201
Concentration camps, Nazi, 50, 125
Control of one's life
  desire for, 76, 77
  fear of losing, 78
  feeling in control, 78, 101–9, 127
    during illness, 107–9
  physical illness and lack of, 101, 102
    asthma, 87, 88. *See also* Hopelessness
Cook-Medley scale, 67, 79
Cooperative ventures, 189–90
Coronary artery bypass operation, 10, 204
Corporate "wellness" programs, 210–11
Corpus callosum, 145
Cortisol (hydrocortisone), 53, 54, 136–37, 138, 139, 142, 148
Cortisol system, 136, 137, 148,149
Cortisone, 136
Costs of health care, 8–9, 204, 214–16
Cousins, Norman, 65–66
Creativity and play, 119–21
Creeps, dealing with, 182
Crisis counseling, on-site, 210
Curiosity, 55, 151, 169
Curren, Kevin, 116
Cushing's syndrome, 53
Cynicism, 79–80, 104

Death. *See* Mortality; Sudden cardiac death
Depression, 51–54, 72, 75, 76, 137, 153, 168

apathy versus, 50, 51
challenges and, 111
exercise and, 193
while in hospital, 107
physical illness and, 52–53, 61, 97, 139, 203
  arthritis, 85
  asthma, 87
  cancer, 59, 61, 162
  death, 92–93
  headaches, 88, 89
  heart attack, 93
  immune system-related disease, 139, 147
  ulcers, 88, 89
response to loss and, 77–78
stress and, 53–54. *See also* Developing a self-healing personality
Developing a self-healing personality, 154–201
  achieving balance, 163–64
  biological coping, 167, 190–99
    biofeedback, 197–98
    exercise, 167, 190–94
    meditation, 195–97
    physical manipulation, 198–99
    systematic relaxation, 167, 194–95
  changing habits slowly, 157–59
  changing thoughts, 174–82
    dealing with creeps, 182
    prioritizing, 181
    self-esteem, 176–77
    success reminders, 174–75
    turning work into play, 180–81
    visual imagery, 178–80
  emotional problems, 168–74
    assessing your personality, 170
    assessing your situation, 170–74
    basic personality patterns, 168–70
  individualizing path toward, 155–56

Developing a self-healing personality (*continued*)

    making time in daily routine, 160–61

    methods that don't work, 154–56, 200–201

    scientific application of psychosocial interventions, 161–63

    selectively altering social environments, 157, 159–60

    social support, 166–67, 190

      buddy system, 188

      cooperative ventures, 189–90

      marriage, 188–89

      in religion, 186–87

      seeking, 185–86

      volunteering, 187–88

    ways of healing, 165–67

      biological means, 167, 190–99

      combinations of, 200

      psychological coping, 166, 174–82

      social relations, 166–67, 183–90

Diabetes, 1, 104, 150–51

Diet, 129–33, 201

Dignity, sense of, 125–26

Disease-prone personalities, 57–97, 133, 137, 143, 151

    blaming the victim, 94–96

    conclusions, 96–97

    failure to replicate, 91–92

    meta-analyses of personality and health, 84–91

    natural-killing cells, 59–60

    overall findings, 91

    psychiatric disorder and mortality, 93–94

    unhealthy motivational states, 75–81. *See also individual diseases*

Divorce, 189

Drugs, treatment of illness with, 205, 219

Duke University, 79

Dunbar, Dr. Flanders, 6–7

Eating habits, 53

    depression and, 52, 54, 168

Emotional inhibition, 147

Emotional training, 112

Endocrine system, 151

    stress and, 32, 33

Endorphin blocker, 144

Endorphins, 144

Enthusiasm, 54–56, 118, 169–70

    survival of cancer and, 60

Environment

    assessing your, 170–74

      at work, 171–73

    control of. *See* Control of one's life

    match between personality and, 42, 74, 99, 170–75

    role of

      in disease, 94, 100, 149

      in personality, 22

Erikson, Dr. Erik, 122

Erikson, Kai, 167

Ethnic differences in response to pain, 17–18

Evaluating new medical developments, 216–19

Exercise, 167, 190–94

    facilities for, funding of, 212

Expectations

    health and, 7–8, 116–18

    Pygmalion effect, 82–83

Extroversion, 56, 58

Failure to replicate, 91–92

Faith healing, 7, 8

Familial hypercholesterolemia, 133

Family, 122–24, 185

Fatigue, 53

Fats in the blood, 150

Fats in the diet, 132–33

    metabolism of, 132, 133, 142

Fear, anticipatory, 165

"Fight or flight" response, 30–31, 32, 46, 53, 147
Finland, study in, 124
Fixx, Jim, 191
Food and Drug Administration, 18
Ford, Gerald, 157
Framingham study, 65, 131, 135
Frankl, Viktor, 125
Franklin, Benjamin, 4, 5, 48, 154, 175
French-Belgian Collaborative Heart Study, 65
Freud, Sigmund, 144–45, 146–47
Friedman, Dr. Meyer, 63
Future of medicine, 219

Galen, 5, 54, 114
Gallstones, 144
Gandhi, Mohandas K., 110, 127
Garza, Felipe, 115
General adaptation syndrome, 35
Genetics and disease, 94
Genetic temperament, 21–23, 47–48
Germs and disease, 33–34, 206–7
Glaser, Dr. Ronald, 149
Glass, Dr. David, 76
Greeks, ancient, 5, 16, 31–32, 48, 54, 79, 96, 97
Grossarth-Maticek, Ronald, 61–62
Gulag Archipelago, The (Solzhenitsyn), 51

Habits, slowly changing, 157–58
Happiness, 55
Hardworking individuals, health of, 72–73, 109–10. *See also* Job stress
Harvard University, 24, 30, 191
Hassles, 41–42
Headaches, 2, 84, 88–89, 151
Health care system in United States, 8–11, 99
 costs of, 8–9, 204, 214–16

emphasis on high technology, 10
economic reward in, 16
neglect of disease prevention, 10, 205
orientation toward curing disease, 99
resistance to change, 206–7
unconscious conspiracy, 204–6
Health insurance, 245
Heart attacks, 23, 38, 148, 162, 194
 counseling victims of, 208
 depression and, 93
 job strain and, 43
 suspiciousness and, 79
 timing of, 40
Heart disease, 1, 2, 23, 39, 40
 cholesterol and, 129–33
 personality and, 61, 63–75, 76, 79, 84, 97, 104
Hepatitis, 150
Hepburn, Katharine, 119, 191
Heroin addicts, 143–44
High blood pressure, 23, 135
High-density lipoprotein (HDL), 137, 142, 143
Hippocrates, 5
Holistic healing, 162
Holmes, Dr. Thomas, 38
Homeostasis of the body, 33–34, 53, 54, 110, 112, 113, 151, 207–8, 219
 ability to recapture, 143–44
 achieving. *See* Developing a self-healing personality
Homicide, 153
Hope, Bob, 4, 5, 17, 98, 114, 127, 180, 198
Hopelessness, 31–32, 43, 50, 76, 77–78
 cancer and, 58, 61, 63
Hormonal system. *See* Endocrine system
Horowitz, Vladimir, 4, 119
Hospices, 123

Hospitals
cost controls, 215, 216
loss of control while in, 107–9
measures to counteract, 107–8
Hostility and aggression, 47–48, 50,
76, 98, 104, 169
exercise and, 193
while in hospital, 107
physical illness and, 97, 104, 203
arthritis, 85
asthma, 87
atherosclerosis, 140–41
heart disease, 67–68, 79, 97. *See
also* Developing a self-healing
personality
Hoxsey, Harry, 116
Hudson, Rock, 149
Humor, sense of, 120, 180–81, 199
Humors, four basic, 5, 32, 54, 96
Hydrocortisone. *See* Cortisol
Hypertension, 23, 135
Hypothalamus, 136, 146

Id, 145
Immigrants, 125
Immune system, 23–24, 34, 49, 53,
97, 130, 137, 138–40, 151,
194
AIDS and, 150
arthritis and, 86
depression and, 139, 147
diabetes and, 151
emotional inhibition and, 147
mood and, 42
natural killer cells, 58–59
stress and, 24, 139–40
Independence, 120, 124
Individual differences, 3–4, 16–19,
24–25, 43–44, 99–100, 119,
129–30
paths toward a self-healing personality and, 155–56
in response to stress, 35–37, 114
Influenza, 150

Inner dissatisfaction, 72
Institute of Medicine, 218
Insulin, 150–51
Internal equilibrium. *See* Homeo-
stasis of the body
Interpersonal relations at work, 74
Interpretation of Dreams, The
(Freud), 144
Introversion and physical illness, 85,
88, 90, 91

Jackson, Jesse, 212–13
James, William, 113
Janis, Irving, 166
Japanese, 110, 124, 183
Job, Book of, 95
Job environment, match between
personality and, 171–73
Job involvement, 73–74
Job stress, 42–43, 74
interpersonal relations and, 74
feeling in control and, 102
Jogging, 167, 190, 191–92
Johns Hopkins University, 22
Precursors Study, 61
Johnson and Johnson, 210–11

Karasek, Dr. Robert, 43
Kelly, Orville, 187–88
Kennedy, John F., 212
Kennedy, Rose Fitzgerald, 120, 191
Kiecolt-Glaser, Dr. Janice, 149
Kimberly-Clark, 211
Kobasa, Dr. Suzanne Ouelette, 103
Kraepelin, Emil, 52
Krebiozen, 7, 8

Laetrile, 7, 8
LaLanne, Jack, 191
Lasser, Terese, 160
Laughter, 199
Lawyers, studies of, 103–5
Leadership promoting physical fit-
ness, 212–13

"Learned Helplessness, Theory of," 77
Levy, Dr. Sandra, 60
Life changes, stress and major, 37–39
Lightner, Candy, 77–78
Limbic system, 146
Lister, Lord, 207
List making, 175
Liver, 150
Lourdes, France, 8, 179
Low-density lipoprotein (LDL), 137, 143, 194
Lown, Dr. Bernard, 24–25
Lung cancer, 60, 149
Lymphocytes, 140

MacLaine, Shirley, 176
McQueen, Steve, 7
Maddi, Dr. Salvatore, 103
Make Today Count, 187, 212
Marriage, 217
    social support from, 166–67, 188–89
Maslow, Abraham, 120
Massage, 198–99
Match between personality and environment, 42, 74, 99, 170–75
Mead, Margaret, 4
Meditation, 167, 195–96
Melancholy. *See* Depression
Melanoma, 58–59
Menninger brothers, 64
Mental rehearsal of solutions to realistic problems, 165
Meta-analyses of personality and health, 3, 84–91
Meta-analysis, 82–84
Metabolism
    disturbed, 130
    of fats, 132, 133, 142
Meyer, Dr. Adolf, 37
Migraines. *See* Headaches
Mistrust, 79

Monkeys, studies with, 140–41
Mortality
    accidents as cause of, 152
    change in philosophy of life of seriously ill, 121
    personality and, 104
    psychiatric disorders and, 93–94
    suicide, 152–53
    will to die, 115
    will to live, 115–19
        emotions linked with, 118–19
Mothers Against Drunk Driving (MADD), 78
Motivational states, unhealthy, 75–81
Multiple sclerosis, 86
Music, 197

Naltrexone, 144
Naps, 196–97
National Academy of Sciences, 218
National Cancer Institute, 60
National Heart, Lung, and Blood Institute, 132
National Institutes of Health, Heart Institute of, 203–4
Natural killer cells (NK cells), 58–59, 139, 194
Negative emotions, 45–54. *See also specific emotions*
Nervous system
    immune system and, 139–40
    neurosis and, 45–46
    stress and, 31, 32–33
    sympathetic, 51, 134–35, 137, 142, 147, 148, 149, 151
Neuroticism, 45–46, 55
New Age movement, 162
New York Times, The, 91
Nonverbal style, 156–57
Norepinephrine (noradrenaline), 48, 135
Nursing home residents, 171

Obesity, 132
On-site crisis counseling, 210
Opiate antagonists, 144
Optimism, 108–9, 165
  realistic, 109
Oregon, 216
Ornish, Dr. Dean, 161–62

Pennebaker, Dr. James, 147
Personality and health, 1–7, 11–29
  disease-prone personalities. *See*
    Disease-prone personalities
  individual differences, 3–5, 16–
    19, 24–25, 43–44
  meta-analyses of, 84–91
  negative emotions. *See* Negative
    emotions
  overall findings, 91
  paths linking, 21–27
    behavior, 25–26
    genetic temperament, 21–23
    misleading links, 26–27
    stress, 23–25
  self-healing personality. *See* Devel-
    oping a self-healing person-
    ality
Pessimism, 78–79
Phlegmatic person. *See* Apathy
Phobics, 47
Phoenix Society, 212
Physical manipulation, 198–99
Physician fees, controlling, 215–16
Physiology, 130
Pituitary, 136
Pituitary-adreno-coritcal axis (cor-
    tisol process), 136, 137, 148,
    149
Placebo effect, 8, 116–18
Play, 119–21, 180–81
Pneumonia, 150
Post-traumatic stress disorder, 47
Poverty and risk of heart disease, 74–
    75
Prayer, 197

Preventive health care, 10, 205, 214
Prioritizing, 181
Promotion of health, cynical atti-
    tudes toward, 27–28
Protective physiological activity, 143
Proverbs, 46, 64
Pryor, Richard, 98
Psychiatric disorders, mortality and,
    93–94
Psychoneuroimmunology, 138, 140
Psychosocial approach to illness, 15,
    18, 29, 37. *See also* Develop-
    ing a self-healing personality;
    Disease-prone personality;
    Self-healing personality; *spe-
    cific illnesses*
Psychosomatic medicine, 3
Pygmalion effect in the classroom,
    82–83

Rabbits, studies of, 142
Radner, Gilda, 94
Rahe, Dr. Richard, 38
Rats, laboratory, 101
Reach to Recovery, 160, 212
Reagan, Ronald, 4, 81
Recreation facilities, public funds
    for, 212
Relaxation, systematic, 167, 194–
    95, 197
Religion, 186–87
"Repetitive strain injury," 18
Repression, 49, 80–81, 145
  apathy and, 49–50, 80–81
  cancer and, 58, 59, 61
Research, evaluating medical, 216–
    19
Responsibility for our own health,
    19–21
Retirement, 72–83
Retirement homes, 171
Rheumatoid arthritis. *See* Arthritis
"Rheumatoid Personality: A Psycho-
    diagnostic Myth, The," 86

Richter, Dr. Curt, 31, 32
Risk factors
    cardiovascular, 203–4
    developing a disease and, 29. *See
        also specific illnesses and risk
        factors*
Rogers, Carl, 119
Roosevelt, Eleanor, 4
Rosenman, Dr. Ray, 63
Rosenthal, Robert, 82–83
Rotter, Dr. Julian, 79–80

Sadness. *See* Depression
Sagan, Carl, 189
Salk, Dr. Jonas, 4, 182
Salutogenesis, theory of, 126
Sanguine personality. *See* Enthu-
    siasm
Sapolsky, Dr. Robert, 141
Sartre, Jean-Paul, 74
Saul, Dr. Leon, 26
Scharansky, Natan, 109
Schopenhauer, Arthur, 111
Schwartz, Dr. Joseph F., 42, 43
Self-absorption, 122
Self-actualization, 120
Self-esteem, 169, 176–77
Self-healing personality, 29, 98–128
    ability to capture one's equilib-
        rium, 143
    coherence, 126
    commitment, sense of, 102–3,
        104–5, 109–10, 127
    creativity and play, 119–21
    definition of, 20
    developing a. *See* Developing a
        self-healing personality
    feeling in control, 101–9, 127
    major types of, 113–15
    multiple brains and, 146
    promoting, 216
    sense of dignity, 125–26
    social ties and social integration,
        121–25, 127

viewing life as a challenge, 103,
    104, 110–13, 127
will to live, 115–19
Self-help peer groups, voluntary,
    211–12
Self-rewards, 175
Seligman, Martin, 77
Selye, Hans, 34–35, 36, 90
Sexual desire, 141–42, 168
Sexual relations, 199
16PF (personality test), 79
Skin cancer, 58–59
Slaney, Mary Decker, 111
Sleep, 52, 53, 54, 168
Smell, sense of, 199
Social environments, selectively al-
    tering, 157, 159–60
Social integration, 121–25, 127,
    166–67
    personality patterns and, 169, 170
    social support, 183–90
        buddy system, 188
        cooperative ventures, 189–90
        marriage, 188–89
        religion, 186–87
        seeking, 185–86
        volunteering, 187–88
Social status and stress, 141–42, 143
Society, social integration in, 124–
    25, 127
Society-wide efforts to improve
    health, 209
Solzhenitsyn, Aleksandr, 51
Spock, Benjamin, 4
Sports, 190, 211
Sterling County, Canada study, 93–
    94
Stress, 23–25, 141–43, 203–4
    basic physiology of, 31–33
    cholesterol level and, 133
    depression and, 54
    development of illness and, 100
    diabetes and, 151
    endocrine system and, 32, 33

Stress (*continued*)
   fight-or-flight response, 30–31, 32, 46, 53, 147
   general stress response, 34–35
   good, 39, 125, 151, 156
   hassles, 41–42
   immune system and, 24, 139
   individual differences in response to, 35–37, 114
   job stress. *See* Job stress
   major life changes and, 37–39
   major types of self-healing personalities and, 114
   match between person and environment, 42, 74, 99, 170–75
   nervous system and. *See* Nervous system
   social integration and, 125
   timing of, 40–41
   ulcers and, 89. *See also* Developing a self-healing personality
Stroke, 1, 2, 135, 146, 148
Subliminal suggestion tapes, 200
Success remedies, 174–75
Sudden cardiac death, 24–25, 32, 110, 135
Sugar in the blood, 150–51
Suicide, 152–53
Superego, 145
Suppression, 49
Surgeon general's reports, 218
Surgery, 205, 219
   recovery from, 165–66
Suspiciousness, 79, 98–99, 103
Sympathetic nervous system, 51, 134–35, 137, 142, 147, 148, 149, 151
Systematic relaxation, 167, 194–95, 197

T cells, 139
Tecumseh, Michigan, study, 80
Testimonials, 218
Testosterone, 142

Times to Remember (Kennedy), 120
Train, John, 105
Trust, 79–80
Type A behavior pattern, 63–66, 76, 162, 193, 208
   description of, 63–64
   evidence linking heart disease and, 65–66
   hostility, 67–68
Type B behavior pattern, 69–72, 143
   description of, 70–71
   phony Type B, 71–72

Ulcers, 1, 2, 84, 86, 89–91,151
   control of one's environment and, 101, 102
Unconscious, 145, 147
Unemployed workers, study of, 106
University of Pittsburgh, 60

Verticular fibrillation, 135
Visual imagery, 178–80
Voice tone, 44, 119, 168
Voluntary self-help peer groups, 211–12
Volunteering, 187–88
"Voodoo death," 31

Washington, George, 6
Walter, Bruno, 197
Washington University School of Medicine, 93
Weight Watchers, 212
Weiss, Dr. Jay, 101
Western Collaborative Group, 65, 67, 162
Western Electric study, 60–61, 162
White, Robert, 106
Will to die, 115
Will to live, 115–19
   emotions linked to, 118–19
Wisdom of the Body, The (Cannon), 207
Wolf, Stuart, 17

Work-site health promotion, 210–11

Work environments, match between personality and, 171–73

Work turned into play, 180–81

Worst-case scenario, 180

Worry, ulcers and, 90

Xerox, 211

Yale University, 57–58

Zborowski, Mark, 17–18